GOD'S GROCERIES
...AS NATURE INTENDED

BY SANDY RODGERS

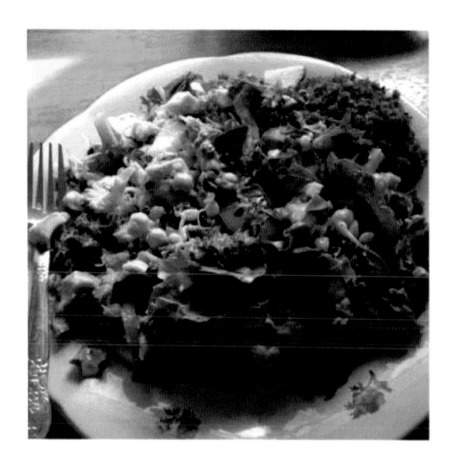

THE MANUAL

GOD's GROCERIES

Presented by

LIFE, LOVE, WELLNESS

SANDY RODGERS MINISTRIES, INC.

SANDY RODGERS AUTHENTIC ASCENSION

DISCLAIMER AND/OR LEGAL NOTICES: The information presented herein represents the view of the author as of the date of publication. Because of the rate with which conditions change, the author reserves the right to alter and update her opinion based on the new conditions. The report is for informational purposes only. While every attempt has been made to verify the information provided in this report, neither the author nor her affiliates/partners, assume any responsibility for errors, inaccuracies or omissions. Any slights of people or organizations are unintentional. If advice concerning legal or related matters is needed, the services of a fully qualified professional should be sought. This report is not intended for use as a source of legal, accounting advice or medical advice. You should be aware of any laws which govern business transactions or other business practices in your country and state. Any reference to any person or business whether living or dead is purely coincidental.

Welcome

It is with extreme appreciation that I welcome you, my friend, to this course. Since my discovery of healing dis-ease, pain and inflammation in the body by simply changing my eating routine and my thinking habits, my desire is to share this wealth of knowledge with the world.

My education has been long and demanding, since the early 1990's, remaining a student always. I have studied under several experts in the field of nutrition, have been certified in Food Healing Science, Plant Based Nutrition and as a Food Educator. I teach at various locations throughout the nation.

In this course you will learn what is meant by the term Whole Food Plant Based Diet (WFPBD). You will receive documented research on the benefits of changing from an animal-protein diet to one of a more natural supply of food. All has been given to us from the beginning by the Creator of all things. We simply need to follow the Master's Plan to live a life filled with well-being and prosperity.

So please come in, take off your coat, and shoes if you like, stay a while and share as we remember together the benefits of:

GOD's GROCERIES

God designed life to be simple… **Rev. Sandy Rodgers**

INTRODUCTION

Over 10,000 years ago our ancestors relied solely on their innate ability to commune with nature. They followed the laws of God and lived according to the seasons. The ancient ones paid attention to the stars, the moon and the sea. They had to rely on the spiritual principles that govern the universe and that kept them healthy. The spirit of man and woman was innately guided by the inner wisdom of the soul.

There is a movement in our healthcare system that is attempting to create more interdependence on medical doctors and the pharmaceutical companies. This is a problem for modern man.

The body, mind and spirit are connected. This is something that the ancient ones knew. We must return to our true selves. The spirit governs the will and where the mind goes energy flows.

We all experience stress in our daily lives. We are affected by stress at work and at home, not to mention the environmental and geopathic stress, i.e. cell phones, computers, microwaves, etc.

In order to maximize your total health you must be all in. In other words you have to do your part. You have to eat right, you have to think right, exercise and rest. You must stay balanced spiritually, this is the way you overcome any challenge in your life. You can't do it half way, if you try you only get half results.

Sandy Rodgers provides a check list for self care. She leads you into a place of forgiveness and gives you seven suggestions that will heal the old wounds. If you do this work you can heal your life. The material in her book will help you become balanced in body, mind and spirit and see results in your life.

These are some of the principles that I've been teaching for over 32 years to my clients. If you follow the nutritional plan and make a commitment to live a healthy and natural life you can heal your life.

The spiritual component cannot be overlooked. Food is medicine and your spirit is your shin and God of the universe dwells within you. So it makes sense that you would eat whole foods. It makes sense that you would avoid fluoride, eliminate the Mercury from your teeth. It makes sense that you would get balanced and you would seek out true health.

The nutritional information and dietary suggestions she shares are medicine to the body and help with a variety of health concerns. **Sandy Rodgers** has overcome several health challenges in her life so this book is about her experiences and there's no better teacher than someone who's overcome.

I'm excited about this book because it shows people the importance of taking responsibility for their own health by being partnered with Source. This book is essential and should be part of everyone's self-care program. Pass it on to your family and friends. It's never too late to heal your body. *God's Groceries... as Nature Intended* is a must read for the 21st century.

The creator of the universe is giving you a garden, now you must take care of it. You start by planting good seeds, eating the right foods. You hydrate with good clean water. You remove the weeds or the negative thinking in your mind.

It's an honor to write this introduction. *God's Groceries... as Nature Intended* is more relevant now than ever. May the readers be a doer of these words. Hippocrates said, "food shall be they medicine." He borrowed from God. Read the book of Genesis.

Mark Armstrong, ND is a practitioner of holistic and alternative modalities/therapies since 1982. He lives and practices in Roswell, Georgia.

TABLE OF CONTENTS

CHAPTER 1

WHY ARE YOU HERE?

SELF- ANALYSIS

MY MOTIVATION

EMOTIONAL RELEASE

SHARING OUR STORIES

God's Groceries pertains to the natural and divine order of life. We must be willing and truthful while doing our self-analysis. It is through our honesty that we shall uncover the reasons why we may stay stuck eating in unhealthy ways. Perhaps eating healthy triggers a family issue for you, or a negative occurrence in your past. Whatever is the reason it is okay. We must recognize and be forthcoming with our self in order to begin the process to living a well-balanced life which begins with good nutrition. So prepare yourself, take a deep breath, and now let it go. Take another deep breath and release. Now the biggest breath yet, hold it, hold it…now release. You should feel a little more relaxed. Now begin.

SELF ANALYSIS

Do you complain often of "feeling bad," and if so, what is the cause?

Do you find fault with other people at the slightest provocation?

Do you deliberately avoid live, healthy foods, and if so, why?

Do you suffer frequently with indigestion? If so, what is the cause?

Does life seem futile and the future hopeless to you? If so, why?

To which do you devote most time, thinking of SUCCESS, or of FAILURE?

Are you gaining or losing self-confidence as you grow older?

Do you learn something of value from all mistakes?

Who has the most inspiring influence upon you? What is the cause?

Do you tolerate negative or discouraging influences which you can avoid?

Are you careless of your personal appearance? If so, when and why?

Have you learned how to "drown your troubles" by being too busy to be annoyed by them?

Would you call yourself a "spineless weakling" if you permitted others, i.e. news, social media, magazines, TV, to do your thinking for you?

Do you neglect internal bathing until auto-intoxication makes you sick, ill-tempered and irritable?

Do you resort to liquor, narcotics, or cigarettes to "quiet your nerves"? If so, why do you not try will-power instead?

Do you have a DEFINITE MAJOR PURPOSE, and if so, what is it, and what plan have you for achieving it?

Have you a method by which you can shield yourself against the negative influence of others?

Do you make deliberate use of auto-suggestion to make your mind positive?

Which do you value most, your material possessions, or your state of health/well-being?

Are you easily influenced by others, against your own judgment?

Has today added anything of value to your stock of knowledge or state of mind?

Do you face squarely the circumstances which make you unhappy, or sidestep the responsibility?

Do you choose, from your daily experiences, lessons or influences which aid in your personal advancement?

Does your presence have a negative or positive influence on other people as a rule?

Have you learned how to create a mental state of mind with which you can shield yourself against all discouraging influences?

Are you conscious of possessing spiritual forces of sufficient power to enable you to keep your mind free from all forms of FEAR?

Does your religion help you to keep your own mind positive?

If you believe that "birds of a feather flock together" what have you learned about yourself by studying the friends whom you attract?

Could it be possible that some person whom you consider to be a friend is, in reality, your worst enemy, because of his negative influence on your mind?

How much time out of every 24 hours do you devote to?

a. your occupation
b. sleep
c. play and relaxation
d. acquiring useful knowledge
e. plain waste
f. Nutrition

What is your greatest worry? Why do you tolerate it?

Do you usually finish everything you begin?

Whom do you believe to be the greatest person living?

Identifying emotional wounds

The first thing we need to do is identify the problem, and realize the need for inner healing. Below is a common list of symptoms for somebody who has an emotional wound:

Inner rawness: there's often a sense of inner rawness and hurt that doesn't seem to go away.

Irritability: it's easy to become irritable with others, even if they aren't doing anything wrong!

Little or no tolerance: there is a low tolerance issue with others, where you expect and demand from them.

Feelings always rising up: feelings of anger, hate, resentment, etc. seem to "rise up" within you at the slightest offense from others.

Overly sensitive about an event in your past: If there are events in your past which cause you to become very sensitive or angry, or even cause you to lash out, then it is likely revealing a deep emotional wound tied in with that event or memory.

Hard to forgive: it becomes very difficult, if not impossible to love and therefore forgive others. It can also be hard to forgive and love yourself. It can even be hard to forgive and love God, even though God has done nothing wrong against you!

Hard to feel loved: it is hard to clearly see and realize the love of others and God in your life. You may be surrounded by people who love you, but it can be difficult to fully feel and receive that love. There seems to be a wall up that blocks the flow of love into your life.

Lashing out: when there's an inner wound that has festered, it becomes easy to lash out or have sudden outbursts of anger, hate, resentment, etc. You may find it easy to lash out at people who love you, and have done you no harm.

Feelings of anger towards God: when a person has been wounded, it becomes easy to blame God for their troubles and hardships. This is the last thing that you want to do when seeking to be healed, because it virtually puts a wall in your mind that can block the healing power of the Holy Spirit to operate. Although God desires to heal your wound, God will not override your free-will, and if you hold hate in your heart against God, it can block efforts to heal your wounds.

Self-hate: many times when a person is hurt from past abuse, they will begin to think that perhaps what happened to them, was deserved because of something they did or the way that they were. This is not true. Abuse is never acceptable, even if a child was being out of order. Parental love disciplines and corrects, but never abuses.

Easily frustrated: because an inner turmoil that an inner wound causes, it is easy to become easily frustrated with everyday chores and responsibilities.

Escapism: as a result of inner turmoil, it is easy to desire to escape or suppress reality. This can be in the form of overeating, drinking, smoking, porn, spending binges, etc. When a person indulges in escapism, addictions can form, and open the door to spirits of addiction, which makes the addictions virtually impossible to break.

Cutting: a person who is a cutter usually has an alter inside the person who is holding much pain, and needs to release the pain or it honestly feels that it deserves the pain (self-hate/religious bondage).

Retaliation urges: because of built-up hate and anger as a result of unforgiveness, somebody who has a festering inner wound will find it easy to retaliate or snap back at those who offend them or step on their toes.

Irresponsible behavior: inner pain has a way of consuming a person's mind, and eventually this can take on a careless approach to life. It is hard to feel good about yourself if you have an inner wound, and if you don't feel good about yourself, it will begin to show in your lifestyle.

Irrational expectations of others: somebody who has been wounded may set high expectations for those around them. They feel that others ought to hold up to unrealistic standards, and are very intolerable to any mistakes made.

Perfectionism: a person who has an emotional wound may also be performance driven. Perhaps they felt like no matter what they did, they could never please a parent or authority figure, and later on in life, that rejection wound causes the person to be a performer to the point where they are never satisfied and burned out by their efforts.

Feelings of hopelessness: This is also a common result of unresolved inner wounds. Since the love of God is blocked in your life, it becomes hard to see why God would love or care for you, and therefore you become an easy target for feelings of hopelessness.

Driven-ness: when you suffer from an emotional wound, it can create a sense of void in your life's meaning, thus driving you to find meaning and purpose and happiness. This could be in the form of college degrees, careers, financial success, etc. Instead of appreciating the person who God has made (YOU!), you find yourself chasing what you think will bring true happiness and purpose to your life.

Obsessive Compulsive Disorder or OCD: Obsessive Compulsive Disorder (OCD) often involves emotional wounds that were never fully healed. This is especially true with people who have bondages to self-hate, self-resentment, self-unforgiveness, etc.

Hostility towards God, self, and others: because of bound up emotions, a person can tend to feel hostile towards God, other people in their life, or even themselves.

This is usually rooted in a form of bitterness against God for not preventing something from happening to you, bitterness against somebody who has wronged or harmed you emotionally, or bitterness against yourself for failures that you've fallen into yourself.

Be honest with yourself!

If you had a headache, would you go to the doctor and tell him, "There's something wrong with me, but I don't want to think about it long enough to figure out what it is! I don't know what's wrong with me! I don't know if it's a headache, a stomachache, a runny nose, or an ingrown toenail!" You would never do that when seeking physical healing, would you? Then why do we so often do this very thing when we are seeking inner healing? We know that there's a problem, a wound, but we don't want to even peek into our pasts to figure out what is really wrong! If you're going to receive healing for an emotional wound, you need to first be honest with yourself and what has happened.

Follow these seven suggestions to heal your wounds:

1. When faced with inner conflict, start by finding your neutrality. Remember all experiences are equal in higher consciousness. Source is meeting your needs, based upon your contributions to energy. You have told Source energetically you want to heal something, and an opportunity has presented itself to you.

2. Love yourself for your vulnerability and humanness. Take time to acknowledge your injury and to source its origins. Don't rush to move away from the uncomfortable feelings. Allow your insight about this wound to rise to your awareness. Give yourself space to feel.

3. Reach for gratitude. Find your humility, and be appreciative for the awareness that you bring into your space. Give thanks for this opportunity. Feed the powerlessness with love and acceptance, either through ritual or some other means of self-support.

4. Be kind to yourself. Don't judge yourself for being wounded. This is a process, not a race. Many of us have layers to uncover to heal the wounds in our space. We can only do as much as we can do. That is enough. There is no timeline you need to meet for anything in your life. Source will always deliver what you need to you.

5. Do not make the mistake of forgetting where your life comes from, the origin of your wealth. The origin of your health. The origin of all the love in your life. Regardless of the vehicle, i.e. job, spouse, family, your needs are being met through your relationship with Source. It is your relationship with Source that determines your abundance.

6. Acknowledge the one-ness of consciousness. There is no *us*, no *them*, only the *one*. Allow the feeling of connection to life to bathe over you. You are one wave in the ocean of life. We are all connected. Everything we do affects everything else. See the God consciousness in you. Recognize that as you heal yourself, you heal the whole. You are mighty and powerful just for being you.

7. Take time to take care of yourself mentally, emotionally, spiritually and physically. This is how you stay connected. It is how you cope with the awareness of your wounds when you see them. It is one big piece in how you gain awareness of your innate wholeness. Finally, ask for insight on how to stay connected to Source. Guess what — you will receive it.

Our goal is not to forget a hurtful event or trauma, but to receive healing for that event, where the Holy Spirit, God, Most High, Universe, Love removes the stinger from it. When we look back upon a healed wound, we can see it in a different way, because it has been healed and is no longer painful to look back upon.

MY MOTIVATION

My first encounter with a health diagnosis of any kind I was in my very early twenties. The grime diagnosis was an Ulcer. Doctor Peter Hershey gently prescribed the newest drug that had hit the market, Tagamet. I valued the advice of this older, kind gentleman who served as my health caregiver. I had no reason not to trust and believe in his professional knowledge. He administered several tests and performed laboratory work on me to determine what was causing my health complaints.

Doctor Hershey explained that the medicine was necessary to correct the problem I was having with indigestion and tenderness in my stomach. I was a dutiful patient and followed the doctor's orders exactly as prescribed. Month after month and year after year I took the Tagamet prescription. My stomach no longer hurt so obviously the pills worked, or so I thought.

However, in my late twenties, I began to experience some rather extreme body acts of elimination. The first incidence was nausea, feeling sick to the stomach all the time. I was not pregnant but it sure felt like it! The sensation was awful, constant and nagging. Next was the headaches. Perhaps I was working too hard and the long steady hours of overtime at work may be finally catching up to me. There must be a reason, I never experienced headaches before. Was this what they called migraines? I was feeling worse every single day. Until suddenly one day at work I was forced to leave and go home...

My body was excreting fluids from every point possible! I was vomiting, had diarrhea and my skin was oozing some form of liquid! I was rushed to the Emergency Room. Upon my admittance the medical staff began performing all the tests to determine the reason for my body to be reacting in this manner. It was horrible! I was given Upper GI, then a lower GI. More X-rays. More pills to take. More of the medical team prodding my body in hopes of making me feel better. Nothing worked and I was still excreting from every pore/opening in my body.

Finally I was blessed to see an Internist. He asked me a series of questions and ended with "What prescriptions do you take?" When I advised him the only one was Tagamet for my ulcer he had this look of relief on his face. His response was, "Stop taking that medicine immediately. It has poisoned your body with heavy metals." So naturally I asked "What should I take for my ulcers? This has been working for me all these years." The Internist boldly replied, "You do not have an ulcer. You have never had an ulcer. If you had an ulcer it would show right here on your x-ray" as he pointed to the machine that displayed my x-rays! The pills that my reliable and trusted Dr. Hershey had advised me to take had MADE ME SICK!!

I had three other such cases of mis-diagnosis from the trusted medical experts. The last two cases that left me searching for alternative methods of healing. I discovered Naturopathic Doctors and the true healer of Raw Food! My diagnosis and grime reports stated I had two irreversible health conditions that required me taking pills the remainder of my life. In the case of the Crohn's Dis-ease I was told if I did not take the pills they would be forced into giving me medical surgery to correct this fatal condition. That was in 2000. I am completely cured of Crohn's Dis-ease. I did not have surgery which was not a guarantee remedy nor did I continue taking the prescription medicine which made me extremely nauseated. I am still alive and well. I did my research, found a reliable Naturopathic Practitioner, Dr. H.H. Worrell and realized perfect health again. Dr. Worrell was so kind and patient with me. I was defending the diagnosis that the allopathic doctor had given me. Dr.

Worrell once told me the only thing that was wrong with me was my absolute faith in the doctors and their false statements. Slowly I began to think a new thought. What if the healing is not what the modern day doctors are concerned with? What if the pills and procedures are not what my body requires to be healthy? What if there is another way to heal? Dr. Worrell said my worst condition was 'Stinking Thinking', believing there was something dreadfully wrong with me.

My mother had shared with me back in the 1980's about herbs and how they can help heal the body of various conditions. She studied and invited me to study with her as she learned the names and ailments the herbs were specifically suited for. I had almost forgotten about this information. I returned to the knowledge of the land, of Mother Earth for answers to health issues. The herbs were not toxic, no added chemicals.

Lastly, I had added so much stress and pressure to my life that my body was ready to explode and implode! I take full responsibility for the condition of my health of that time. I had over-burdened my sensitive balance. Willingly placed myself under tremendous strain of several major-portioned events in a short time frame, of which I was a key player in each situation. A family reunion, asking family members to return to our place of origin. Successfully researching and documenting the family roots. Traversed the back country trails and roads to uncover certain family truths that had been buried and forgotten about. A major Energy Healers Retreat of which I served as Project Manager, pulling all the resources together to host this debut affair. Hosting my own Wholistic Wellness Fair to bring awareness of alternative modalities to the community. This is but a brief recollection of the major unfolding's for an 18 month period in my life that took a toll and rocked me off my feet, literally.

My last health opportunity was called Psoriasis with Eczema mixed with Venus Stasis. My feet, ankles and legs were swollen so bad I was unable to wear regular shoes for months. My hands, wrists and arms were a holy mess as well. Large red spots, swollen and non-stop itching. The skin rash was spreading unto my chest, my back, upper legs and it was traumatic! Above all the holistic remedies and treatments I were advised to try, I was still experiencing the spread of this awful and painful condition. That was the exact moment that I found my way to Living Foods Institute in Atlanta. There I learned how to eat and prepare RAW FOOD DISHES!! Since the completion and continuation of consuming a Whole Food Plant Based Diet my body is completely restored to health and vitality along with shedding a few pounds along the way.

As people saw my recovery take place they would ask what and how did I manage to cure this incurable dis-ease. When I would explain my journey they would began asking me questions about their own health issues. It was paramount for me to share this information with people. I do and as often as possible provide people with the resources they need to educate themselves on healthier alternatives to healing and maintaining their health.

The ladies at L.A. Fitness, where I am a regular member are my biggest cheerleaders in insisting I teach classes and provide this uncommon knowledge to folks like them. Many want me to help their parents who have become victims of this overburdened society of pill popping.

So to the members of L.A. Fitness in Austell Georgia who said; "We are waiting. When are you going to open your own wellness center?" Here is the beginning, a course dedicated to wellness.

EMOTIONAL MAKE OVER

Tips for Emotional Healing
What really helps us reduce our sadness, anxiety, and other emotional distress?

When my granddaughter was a small child and we were having one of our heart to heart conversations she said, "Grandma Sandy – There is no such thing as depression. The person just needs their laugh box filled up!!" Out of the mouths of babes. She was young and being sad and down was not an option to her. I still love the simplicity of her statement.

So what is your state of mental wellness? Yes we each have our turn at some negative energy stirring around in us. The question here is how long do you allow it to be a guest in your consciousness? Do you fill your laugh box or chose to settle for depression? Somewhere along this journey of life, we heard that life is supposed to be easy and without any discomfort. We must have because there are far too many individuals who are mad and upset that they get to experience life in all its wonder and amazement. They literally ask themselves and others too, what did I do wrong?? Why am I being dealt this terrible hand?

When an outsider looks to assist, they do not see the same misfortune as the teller of the gloom and doom story. What helps relieve this distress? What helps a person to heal? What helps is a reality based on real life circumstances. When we can take the sting out of the situation, it allows the person to view it from another perspective perhaps not so gloom and doom as they once saw it.

Suggestions to fill your laugh box:
1. Be you
You must be yourself. I have a friend who is comfortable with her weight although some would criticize her for being 'thick.' She says 'Cute in the face and thick in the waist. Beautiful either way.' Be 'In Love' with you however you are right now! Honoring and respecting the person you currently are means that you are whole and complete. No wishing or hoping to be someone else. YOU are more than enough. Love YOU.

2. Create yourself
Do you desire to change any attribute about who you are? Transformation takes courage and commitment. Who are you? Are you living someone else's version of you? You are created as unique and awesome as anyone. YOU are an unrepeatable miracle. So what does that mean to you? You come with attributes, capacities and abilities. Your family of origin nor your environment can predict your fullness of expression. Can you envision the person you truly desire to be? Ask yourself *"who do I want to be?"* **And honestly answer from only your viewpoint. Opinions of others is NOT YOUR BUSINESS OR CONCERN!!**

3. LOVE is Everything

I co-wrote this song with my nephew, Anthony AK King. Actually it's his song and I assisted him with adding a few of my words. Participating with this project gave me another opportunity to look at life differently. What if...*LOVE IS EVERYTHING?* How wild and wonderful would our lives be? We would live so completely naturally. Happy, free and unrestricted. AS LOVE reside in our soul and spirit, we ooze a calming elixir out into the atmosphere. Not only are we calm but we help others around us to be calm and serene also. Get the song @ www.anthonyakking.com CD **Love Is Everything.**

4. Can you do this another way?

Our thoughts determine our outcome and our outlook. Our thoughts color and shape our reality. It is simply how you think that determines what is projected onto the screen of your life. Who is a part of your movie cast? Who has the starring role? Who is the Director? The supporting cast? Who is creating the music score? Our thoughts are so powerful. Changing our thoughts is not a difficult task. Just Do It...

5. Forgive the past

The past is over and done with. The only thing we can change about the past is how we choose to look and remember it. In my workshop "FORGIVENESS" I ask the participants to choose to look at the relationship, the situation with absolute eyes of love. To honor whatever happened and again choose to look at it through the eyes of love and acceptance. There is no one perfect way to do or be, we each have choices and may opt to handle the same situation differently. Give yourself and others permission to move forward in forgiveness and love.

6. Flip the happy switch ON!

We release the need to be a victim or a person who moans and groans through life. Instead we happily anticipate joyous endings to all the activities we engage in. We decide to switch the HAPPY button on. We celebrate all of life. Not just those parts we describe as being 'good' ones but even the ones we call not so good. In the end, "It's all Good, all the time!" and this too shall pass. Even if you do not believe it is possible just try it for now. You have nothing to lose. **Just flip the happy switch.**

7. Make new goals

Decide on a daily basis that you will wake up and be excited about the presence of a new day. Be happy that you can design your life and future. Our emotional life is so real. I remember my Psychiatrist Dr. Robert Schmidt once told me that just because you cannot see the emotional wounds does not make them any less important to our overall health and well-being. He advised me if I had a broken leg in a cast that would probably signal to me it was okay to take care of it. But the same thing is true for our mental health also. We know when we are off. Take care to honor you and be good to yourself at all times.

8. Set your boundaries

You can decide that the boundaries you set are worth the respect from others. Determine what your boundaries are. Experiment with grounding and connecting to the Source of your understanding. You may call It - God, Allah, Buddha, Father, Lord, or you may not believe in a Master Energy Source at all. Either way is perfectly okay. Grounding allows you to make connection and connect with the Life Force Energy of the Universe. You can literally feel the intense positive energy radiating up through your body. From the balls of your feet up to the crown of your head. Allow it to just BE there with you. This practice will allow you to set boundaries more clearly because you know what it feels like. That connection you got from BE-ing with Mother Earth is your boundary. Do not allow others to disrupt it.

9. Upgrade your barometer of life

Choose to see life as a positive force. When and if you do not welcome or feel positive, fully experience the emotions and allow them to pass. Honoring all of your emotions alerts your mental self you are dedicated to treating everything equally. The ego does get to beat you up because you have missed the mark you set for yourself. The ego also does not boasts that you surpassed a goal. Set your intention to be your best and celebrate you.

10 Being in Balance

Being in balance is perhaps the best place to be. You get to set the balance bar. What will you include, family, work, interpersonal relationships, relaxation, physical fitness, healthy living, energetic balance or what? What do you believe is the optimal life balance? You do know what is right for you. Others may attempt to interfere and offer you advice but always know that you are your best advice source.

We always have a choice. Sometimes making the choice is a major undertaking. Takes a great deal of courage. We forget we **can** control our destiny. We forget we have the power. We now choose to remember our strength and our courage. We accept each incidence as a gift to our growth and wellbeing. We know it has come to bless and not curse us. Life is grand and living it fully is the greatest acknowledgement of our choices.

Author Eric Maisel states *"Who knows if we are in the throes of a "new depression epidemic" or a "new anxiety epidemic" or whether keen emotional distress has been a significant feature of human existence from the beginning. What is different now is that the paradigm of self-help is completely available to anyone who would like to reduce his or her emotional distress. You can understand yourself; you can form intentions and carry them out; you can learn from experience; you can grow and heal. Naturally none of this is true if you are unwilling to do the work required. But if you are, you have an excellent chance of reducing your emotional distress and experiencing genuine emotional health."*

SHARING OUR STORIES

It is imperative that we tell our story. Not for anything other than to validate who you are. You are a valuable, loveable, worthy, miracle waiting for self-expression.

Oftentimes the only obstacle blocking us from receiving of the vast abundance God has for us is accepting our 'value and self-worth.'

Learning Value in Our Story
©2007 Sandy Rodgers Ministries

Often times the only obstacle blocking us from receiving of the vast abundance God has for us is accepting our 'value and worth.'

Many have been led to deny their story, by hearing 'keep your business to yourself', or similar phrases. Or perhaps you discounted your feelings because you heard, 'things aren't that bad.'

We hear powerful and amazing sermons, attend top-rated seminars and yet somehow we feel things just are not changing in our life.

It's time to tell your story, to validate your worthiness and open yourself to receive ALL that God has – just for YOU! Once we own our feelings, whatever they are now or have been in the past, we receive grace. When we know we are whole, complete and healthy children of God, we can tell our story proudly. We know that God has brought us through to this moment to serve as a blessing to ourselves and others. Our trials, tribulations and subsequent victories prepared us for who we are today. The past is gone, Thanks God.

Accepting our true nature of 'goodness', we can fully receive and apply the prosperity lessons we are learning. We say 'Yes' to God and ourselves. Go ahead and give yourself liberty to tell your story. You can write it out. You can share within a safe environment, a loving support group or trusted friend.

You may even find while sharing that your story is the same as another. We are each a part of the 'One Family of God.'

Doing this exercise during my weekly sessions within the HIV/AIDS community has brought new life springing forth from these individuals who had accepted they were no good and good for nothing. As we each share our story healing has taken place in wondrous ways. The group is extremely supportive and encourages each other to tell the whole story. So we share about drug use and abuse. We tell about our childhood horrors of being molested or raped. We share from a place of safety knowing the others will still embrace us with unconditional love. We trust and know that our past is just that, over and done with. That the past is something we cannot change. We then place total forgiveness around the situation and persons involved, including and most importantly ourselves. We proceed to wrap the situation and people in absolute love. Lives are changing. New life is ever present. The individuals are currently doing things that they thought were impossible. They are going back to school to learn a new trade, computer skills; careers in the medical field among others. Moving out from the shelters into their own homes is another result. This is happening because they have been freed from the shackles of their past. They have allowed a new thought to be entertained in their memory and hearts. Our stories are real and worthy to be told. You are worthy and deserve to live a full life void of unforgiveness and bitterness. It is possible to release, forgive and love any and all unpleasant situations from your past. It is now time to live life fully in harmony and joy.

Whatever is holding you back from fully experiencing life, remember it, forgive it and then love it! This is the way to a wonderful life experience here on earth. Your story is whatever you say it is, it does not have to be true for anyone other than yourself. So tell it. Celebrate your victory over the past. Honor exactly where you are this very day and LIVE!

Watch miracles unfold as you lovingly embrace your awesome, wonderful self.

Remember, I Love You.

Rev. Sandy Rodgers

CHAPTER 2

SELF-CARE

SPIRITUAL SELF

CHANGE/ACCEPTANCE

SELF-CARE

Self-care is the unconditional assuming responsibility of one's well-being. Many self-care rituals can be performed in the privacy of one's residence, if desired. Self-care literally means that you take care of you! Self-care cannot be transferred to someone else to do for you. Self-care is essential to a high quality of life and living.

I am attaching various resources to help along this field of self-care. You can always find additional activities to engage in.

A LIST OF SELF-CARE ACTIVITIES

GROUNDING EXERCISES –
Grounding exercises are a way for you to firmly anchor yourself in the present.
Grounding exercises are about using our senses (see, hear, smell, taste, touch) to build our mind and body connection in the present. In working through the grounding exercises suggested here, you might find one or two that work for you – remembering only to use the exercises that you feel comfortable with.

EXERCISES AND STRETCHING
Find routines online if you desire to do in the privacy of your home. Join a gym, do yoga, become a part of a fitness community. Upon awakening stretch UP to heaven and give thanks! Begin the day in Gratitude while flexing your muscles....

SUNSHINE –
Go outside and bask in the sunlight. The Sun is the only true source of Vitamin D! We are gifted with the natural ingredients to live a healthy life. The gifts are from the Source of All Life!
The best times to sunbathe is early morning or late afternoon. Get at least 15 – 30 minutes daily for optimum health benefits.

THE BIG LIST OF SELF-CARE ACTIVITIES

Check the ones you are willing to do, and then add any activities that you can think of:

___ Talk to a friend on the telephone
___ Go out and visit a friend
___ Invite a friend to come to your home
___ Text message your friends
___ Organize a party
___ Exercise
___ Lift weights
___ Do yoga, tai chi, or Pilates, or take classes to learn
___ Stretch your muscles
___ Eat your favorite ice cream
___ Go for a walk in a park or someplace else that's peaceful
___ Go get a haircut
___ Sleep or take a nap
___ Go outside and watch the clouds
___ Go jog
___ Ride your bike
___ Go for a swim
___ Go hiking
___ Do something exciting like surfing, rock climbing, skiing, skydiving, motorcycle riding, or kayaking, or go learn how to do one of these things
___ Go to your local playground and join a game being played or watch a game
___ Buy something on the internet
___ Go play something you can do by yourself if no one else is around, like basketball, bowling, handball, miniature golf, billiards, or hitting a tennis ball against the wall
___ Get out of your house, even if you just just sit outside
___ Plan a trip to somewhere you've never been before
___ Go to a spa
___ Go to a library
___ Go to a bookstore and read
___ Go to your favorite café for coffee or tea
___ Visit a museum or local art gallery
___ Go to the mall or the park and watch other people; try to imagine what they're thinking
___ Pray or meditate
___ Go to your church, synagogue, temple, or other place of worship
___ Join a group
___ Write a letter to your higher power

___ Cook your favorite dish or meal
___ Cook a recipe that you've never tried before
___ Take a cooking class
___ Go out for something to eat
___ Go outside and play with your pet
___ Go borrow a friend's dog and take it to the park
___ Give your pet a bath

___ Go outside and watch the birds and other animals
___ Find something funny to do, like reading the Sunday comics
___ Visit fun Web sites and keep a list of them
___ Watch a funny movie (start collecting funny movies to watch when you're feeling overwhelmed)
___ Go to the movies
___ Watch television
___ Listen to the radio
___ Go to a sporting event, like a baseball game
___ Play a game with a friend
___ Play solitaire
___ Play video games
___ Go online to chat
___ Visit your favorite Web sites
___ Go shopping
___ Do a puzzle with a lot of pieces
___ Sell something you don't want on the internet
___ Create your own Web site
___ Join an internet dating site
___ Buy something on the internet
___ Get a massage
___ Go for a drive in your car or go for a ride on public transportation
___ Eat chocolate (it's good for you!) or eat something else you really like
___ Sign up for a class that excites you at a local college, adult school or online
___ Read your favorite book, magazine or newspaper
___ Read a trashy celebrity magazine
___ Write a letter to a friend or family member
___ Write things you like about yourself on paper
___ Write a poem, story, movie or play
___ Write in your journal
___ Write a loving letter to yourself when you're feeling good and keep it with you to read when you're feeling upset

___ Call a family member you haven't
     Spoken to in a long time
___ Learn a new language
___ Sing or learn how to sing
___ Play a musical instrument or learn
     how to play one
___ Write a song
___ Listen to some upbeat, happy music
     (start making a collection to play when
     You're feeling upset)
___ Turn on some loud music and dance
___ Memorize lines from your favorite movie,
     play or song
___ Make a movie or video
___ Take photographs
___ Join a public-speaking group and
     write a speech
___ Participate in a local theatre group
___ Sing in a local choir
___ Plant a garden
___ Work outside
___ Knit, crochet, or sew—learn how to
___ Make a scrapbook with pictures
___ Paint your nails
___ Trim your nails
___ Change your hair color
___ Take a bubble bath or shower
___ Work on your car, truck, motorcycle or bicycle

___ Make a list of ten things you're good at or like
     about yourself and keep it with you to read when
     you're feeling upset
___ Draw a picture
___ Paint a picture with a brush or your fingers
___ Make a list of the people you admire and describe
     what it is you like about them
___ Write a story about the craziest or funniest thing
     that has ever happened to you
___ Make a list of ten things you would like to do
     before you die
___ Write a letter to someone who has made your life
     better and tell them why (you don't have to send
     the letter if you don't want to)
___ Create your own list of self-care activities
___ Other ideas: _____
     _____
     _____
     _____
     _____
     _____

Note: Adapted from *The Dialectical Behavior Therapy Skills Workbook*. McKay et al. 2007 p. 15

GROUNDING

Grounding is a way of helping yourself cope with stressful periods in your life. While the intrusive symptoms of traumatic stress – like flashbacks, memories, and upsetting thoughts – cannot always be stopped, you can learn techniques that will minimize their impact. Grounding techniques can help you regain a sense of safety and control in your life. They can help you anchor yourself in the here and now and keep you from getting lost in the past.

Below you will find a description of several grounding techniques. ** One (or more) of these techniques is likely to suit you better than the others. Choose the technique that you would like to focus on and practice it regularly, especially when you are feeling well. If you become good at using the technique during non-crisis times, you will be better equipped to use it when you are in crisis.

Seated Grounded Posture: This is a posture in which both feet are on the floor and your spine is straight, but not rigidly so. In this posture, you are actively aware of your body's existence and its connection to the ground. Your legs should be uncrossed – this allows the flow of energy to pass freely through the body. Your hands may be resting on your thighs or on the arms of the chair. Your head is held high. Notice the way your body rests in the chair; notice the way your feet are resting on the ground. This is a posture that can allow you to feel both strong and at ease.

Mindful Walking: Walk carefully, mindfully around the room. Mindful walking can be slow or brisk. The goal is to be fully present with each step as you take it. Bring your attention to the actual sensations of walking. Notice how the heel, then the ball of your foot makes contact with the floor as you walk. Notice the bend in your knees, the flex in your toes, and the shift in your weight with each step you take. When your attention wanders, bring it back to your walking. Center yourself in your body and be present in the moment. Count ten steps, and ten more, and ten more, until you feel calmed.

Writing / Saying Grounding Statements: Develop several grounding statements that remind you that you are safe and provide you with comfort. You may want to write the statements on a small piece of paper or "flashcard" and carry them around in your wallet. You may want to write the statement on a larger piece of paper that you will hang on a wall in your home. Write your statements in a color that represents safety and strength to you. You can say the statements out loud, or simply read or think them.
Examples of grounding statements include:
 • "This feeling will soon pass."
 • "You are no longer a child. You are an adult now, and you are safe."
 • "You are strong, you are safe now."
Develop your own grounding statements, ones that have special meaning for you.

Grounding through Breathing: The breath serves wonderfully as a focus for your attention. Think of it as an anchor that holds you in the present moment and guides you back to the here and now when your mind wanders to the past. By bringing awareness to your breathing, you are reminding yourself that you are here now. Breathe in and attend to the feeling of breathing in; breathe out and attend to the feeling of breathing out. You may want to focus on the air coming in and out of your nostrils or on your abdomen expanding and contracting as you breathe. You may want to count ten breaths on the exhale, and keep counting groups of ten breaths until you feel calmed. You may also want to use calming, grounding statements as you breathe, like:

• **Inhaling,** "I am breathing in calm." or "I am breathing in good energy."
• **Exhaling,** "I am breathing out anxiety," or "I am breathing out bad energy," or "I am safe."

Other Grounding Techniques
- Dance and/or sing to a song that makes you feel good.
- Stamp your feet. Feel the power in your legs.
- Visual grounding
- Make eye contact with a safe person.
- Scan the room to remind yourself that you are here now.
- Don't direct your gaze downward. Look up, look out, look around.
- Hold, look at, listen to and/or smell a grounding object.

Grounding objects may be distinguished by their smell, shape, weight, sound, or texture. Any object that comforts you, that helps you to remember that you are in the present, rather than the past, can be a grounding object.
Some examples are:
- A smooth stone that you've found on the beach
- A bell that, when you ring it, has a soothing sound
- A piece of sandpaper with a course texture
- A photograph of a beautiful scene or of loved ones
- A small vial of a pleasant fragrance
- A piece of jewelry, like a ring or bracelet
- A picture that you've drawn of a scene that represents safety and comfort.

You may want to hold, look at, smell, listen to your grounding object while engaged in one of the other grounding techniques. For example, you can hold your stone while repeating your grounding statements, while walking mindfully, or while doing grounding breathing. This way, you strengthen the grounding properties of your grounding object because it becomes associated with other experiences of comfort and safety. If your grounding object is small enough, you can carry it with you wherever you go. Knowing that you have access to a small oasis of calm and comfort right there can help.

Courtesy: Dr. Patti Levin www.drpattilevin.com

Exercise & Physical Activity: Your Everyday Guide from the National Institute on Aging

Sample Exercises - Flexibility

How easy is it for you to turn around and look behind you before backing out of a parking space? What about bending down to tie your shoes? Flexibility exercises will help you do both more easily!

How to Improve Your Flexibility

Stretching, or flexibility, exercises are an important part of your physical activity program. They give you more freedom of movement for your physical activities and for everyday activities such as getting dressed and reaching objects on a shelf. Stretching exercises can improve your flexibility but will not improve your endurance or strength.

How Much, How Often

- Do each stretching exercise 3 to 5 times at each session.

- Slowly stretch into the desired position, as far as possible without pain, and hold the stretch for 10 to 30 seconds. Relax, breathe, then repeat, trying to stretch farther.

Safety

- Talk with your doctor if you are unsure about a particular exercise. For example, if you've had hip or back surgery, talk with your doctor before doing lower-body exercises.

- Always warm up before stretching exercises. Stretch after endurance or strength exercises. If you are doing only stretching exercises, warm up with a few minutes of easy walking first. Stretching your muscles before they are warmed up may result in injury.

- Always remember to breathe normally while holding a stretch.

- Stretching may feel slightly uncomfortable; for example, a mild pulling feeling is normal.

- You are stretching too far if you feel sharp or stabbing pain, or joint pain — while doing the stretch or even the next day. Reduce the stretch so that it doesn't hurt.

- Never "bounce" into a stretch. Make slow, steady movements instead. Jerking into position can cause muscles to tighten, possibly causing injury.

- Avoid "locking" your joints. Straighten your arms and legs when you stretch them, but don't hold them tightly in a straight position. Your joints should always be slightly bent while stretching.

Reference: https://www.nia.nih.gov/health/publication/exercise-physical-activity/sample-exercises-flexibility

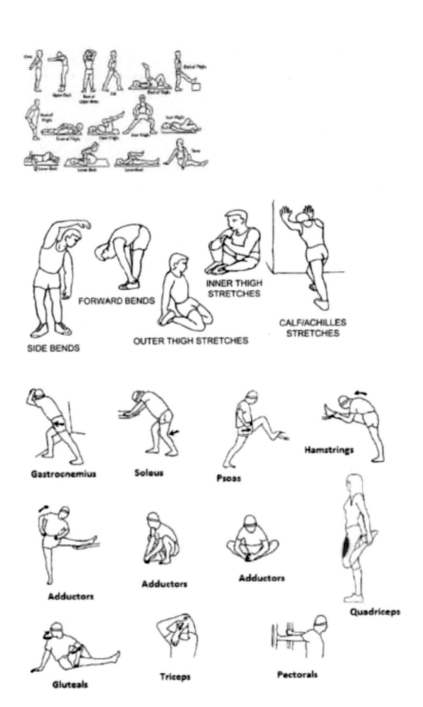

SIDE BENDS

FORWARD BENDS

INNER THIGH STRETCHES

OUTER THIGH STRETCHES

CALF/ACHILLES STRETCHES

Gastrocnemius

Soleus

Psoas

Hamstrings

Adductors

Adductors

Adductors

Quadriceps

Gluteals

Triceps

Pectorals

DESK STRETCHES

- Breathe easily
- No bouncing or forcing
- No pain!
- *Feel* the stretch
- Relax
- See Stretching Instructions, pp. 77–84

5
5 sec.
p. 84

9
10 sec.
p. 82

1
5 sec., 3 times
p. 82

6
5 sec.
each side
p. 84

10
10 sec.
p. 81

2
5 sec., 3 times
p. 82

7
5 sec.
p. 84

11
5 sec.
each side
p. 82

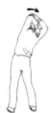

3
5 sec., 2 times
p. 81

8
10 sec.
each arm
p. 81

12
10 sec.
p. 79

4
5 sec., 2 times
p. 84

- Prolonged sitting at a desk or computer terminal can cause muscular tension and pain.
- Taking a few minutes to do a series of stretches can make your whole body feel better.
- Learn to stretch spontaneously throughout the day whenever you feel tense.
- Don't just do seated stretches, but do some standing stretches too. Good for circulation.

From the book:

34 **Getting in Shape** © 2002 Shelter Publications, Inc.   **www.shelterpub.com**   *Photocopy this page and keep it in your desk drawer.*

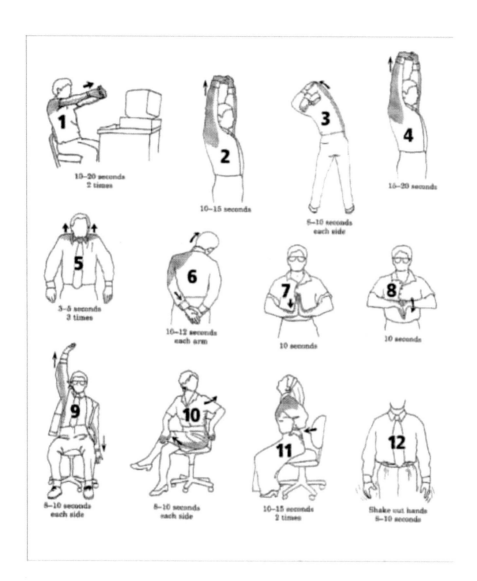

1
10–20 seconds
2 times

2
10–15 seconds

3
8–10 seconds
each side

4
15–20 seconds

5
3–5 seconds
3 times

6
10–12 seconds
each arm

7
10 seconds

8
10 seconds

9
8–10 seconds
each side

10
8–10 seconds
each side

11
10–15 seconds
2 times

12
Shake out hands
8–10 seconds

SPIRITUAL SELF

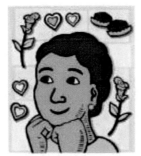

HEART MEDITATION

Once a day, sit quietly and place your hands upon your heart. Send it Love and allow yourself to feel the love your heart has for you. It has been beating for you since before you were born and will work for you as long as you choose to live. Look into your heart and see if there is any bitterness or resentment lingering there. Gently wash it away with forgiveness and understanding. If you could but just see the larger picture, you would understand the lessons. Send love to each member of your family and forgive them. Feel your heart relaxing and being at peace. Your heart is Love and the blood in your veins is Joy. Your heart is now lovingly pumping joy throughout your body. All is well and you are safe.

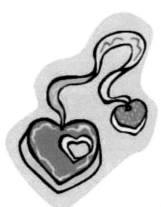

*The missing piece is **<u>FORGIVENESS</u>!!!***

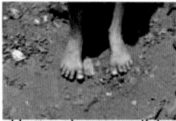

Do you notice you feel better when you walk barefoot on the Earth? Recent research has explained why this happens.

Your immune system functions optimally when your body has an adequate supply of electrons, which are easily and naturally obtained by barefoot contact with the Earth.

Research indicates that electrons from the Earth have antioxidant effects that can protect your body from inflammation and its many well-documented health consequences. For most of our evolutionary history, humans have had continuous contact with the Earth.

There is an emerging science documenting how conductive contact with the Earth, which is also known as Earthing or grounding, is highly beneficial to your health and its completely safe. Earthing appears to minimize the consequences of exposure to potentially disruptive fields like "electromagnetic pollution" or "dirty electricity."

Grounding or Earthing is defined as placing one's bare feet on the ground whether it be dirt, grass, sand or concrete (especially when humid or wet). When you ground to the electron-enriched earth, an improved balance of the sympathetic and parasympathetic nervous system occurs.

Modern science has thoroughly documented the connection between inflammation and all of the chronic diseases, including the diseases of aging and the aging process itself. It is important to understand that inflammation is a condition that can be reduced or prevented by grounding your body to the Earth, the way virtually all of your ancestors have done for hundreds if not thousands of generations.

Author: Dr Mercola

GROUNDED BOUNDARIES

GUIDED MEDITATION

ACTIVITY

When we connect with "Mother Earth" something happens that heals our bodies. We feel the "Oneness" of all life and existence. We are ONE.

Honor YOU! Feel the power of the earth beneath your feet. This may seem unfamiliar to you, but not long ago children walked barefooted as they joyously played outside. In our modern world we seldom see this and certainly do not recommend our children do this. But this exercise is for YOU. Please take off your shoes and choose to walk barefoot.

What does this activity taste like? That's correct 'taste'. Perhaps you feel a sensation that comes up from the earth into your body that you have not felt before. Use a different human sense/function than you would normally. How do you feel? Do you sense the connection? Can you taste it?

This boundary is your personal connection with your Soul and Spirit. Within this unity you are safe and protected. You are Loved and Valued. This is your sacred spot. This is where you are and can be all that you desire.

In this setting we will explore how to establish your personal boundaries with all others. You will understand the importance of always honoring your sacred space. No person is allowed to violate you or your boundaries. It is YOUR connection with Infinite Source, God, Holy Spirit, Universe, Most High.

There is a sacredness when you 'feel' and 'taste' Mother Earth. You know you belong to a most all-inclusive family. Love is the center. Harmony is the outer and Peace is woven in every fabric.

What is Energy Medicine?

Energy Medicine is a new field with ancient origins, a field that is opening new avenues of support both for individuals experiencing health challenges and for medical practitioners seeking to support their patients' healing in less invasive ways.

To quote Dr. Mehmet Oz recently on the Oprah Winfrey Show, "Energy medicine is the future of all medicine. We're beginning now to understand things that we know in our hearts are true but we could never measure. As we get better at understanding how little we know about the body, we begin to realize that the next big frontier in medicine is energy medicine. It's not the mechanistic part of the joints moving. It's not the chemistry our body – its understanding for the first time how energy influences how we feel."

Energy Medicine recognizes energy as a vital living force which penetrates, supports and organizes all Life, and is, in fact, essential to the maintenance of all Life. The practice of energy medicine focuses on optimizing the flow and balance of this vital living force as the very foundation of human well-being. Energy Medicine draws from hundreds of traditional healing methods. It integrates ancient knowledge with modern perspectives and new technologies. And it is at once both a complement to traditional medical treatment and a complete self-help and self-care system. Energy Medicine technologies and techniques today include – but are not limited to – herbology and botanical medicine, homeopathy, Reiki, light and magnet therapy, color therapy, Therapeutic Touch, Cranial Sacral Therapy, bio-field therapy, holistic remedies of many kinds, subtle energy infusion technologies, energy psychology, Traditional Chinese Medicine, Ayurvedic Medicine, acupuncture, yoga, Tai Chi, Qigong. In these increasingly challenging times, innovative energy medicine tools and techniques can help the average person and the skilled health practitioner work better to optimize both the energy fields in the body and the body's chemical and biological systems, thereby solving complex health challenges in ways that are less toxic and less invasive to the body than traditional medicine now has to offer. Energy Medicine is rapidly contributing to a whole new way to look at health and healthcare. It is our hope that it may soon transform global healthcare systems into systems of wellness – rather than systems of illness.

Dr. Oz featured Reiki as a complementary therapy on his 1/6/09 show

Dr. Oz is a renowned cardiac surgeon at one of the top teaching hospitals in the world, and he would not give his attention to anything risky or without merit. In fact, he was the first to let Julie Motz, a Reiki Practitioner, in the OR with him to administer Reiki treatments during cardiac surgery back in the 1980's.

We will practice some simple Reiki hand placements in the conference/training session. If you are not in attendance of a live class, please email for additional information on securing a Reiki Practitioner at srm@sandyrodgersministries.org .

Sit quietly and allow yourself to relax. You may say a prayer or do affirmations, simply become at peace. Close your eyes for a short period and continue to relax more and more. Gently rub your hands together. Feel your life-force energy circulating between your hands. You are feeling the energy that is always present, yet we take for granted or do not realize its gift to us. As you become aware of this YOUR energy, get to know it and feel it. This is your spiritual energy. Now take and place your hands over your eyes. You will feel a deep sensation flowing through your eyelids to the pupil. Allow your hands to rest there for s moment. Next move your hands to your ears. Cup your hands over both ears. Again allow your hands to rest there for a while. You can this at any time you want to calm nervous tension or just want to renew the energy inside of your body temple.
We are powerful energy centered humans. We have the means to heal ourselves by simple touch of our own hands. How awesome is this gift to us from The Creator.

SAVING ELDERS
Rev. Sandy Rodgers, CRMT

The title is mis-leading mainly because we cannot save anyone. We can assist others along their path to quality care of themselves but never save. Our American health care, which is more of a sick-care system, does little if anything to aide individuals to creating for themselves a healthy or healthier lifestyle. We seem to thrive on sickness and not wellness!

As we become a more mature nation, baby-boomers being the largest population, it stands to reason that our focus would be on establishing ways to help those be and/or live a richer life. When taken from a theological perspective, scripture assures us that Jesus came to demonstrate our human power, and we could have more than what he had.

When we look at our behavior from a historical view, we understand that our ways must improve and become more advanced as the society makes monumental strives forward. We are more than we were in the last decade, and much more advance than we were two decades ago.

Taking a medical glance, in ancient times Doctors were only paid when the patient remained well. When the person became ill, it was considered the Doctor had not fulfilled their obligation therefore payment was withheld. In a more recent time, we knew how to gather herbs and roots from our gardens or the woods to mix and create a concoction that would cure whatever the ailment was.

As medical science has expanded, new medications generated in the laboratories, research not given sufficient time to test their effects on humans, our society is now plagued with a large portion of the population being prescribed pills to combat the illness. However it seems there is always a price to pay for these quick-fix remedies. Loss of life, loss of body parts and other such losses as reported on the television with numerous advertisements offering monetary compensation if you experienced a negative reaction while taking the prescription given to you by the doctor.

Sad as this may sound to you, it gets worse with our elder population. Our seniors are covered medically by the government, Medicare. If you were not aware you would think this gives the medical professional a green light to order and prescribe any number of medications to our senior citizens. As a society we now accept the notion that at a particular age we must be taking some kind of medicine to stay well! I find this absurd, yet very true.

As for myself, when I went to have a regular medical checkup and was asked which medications I take, as I said 'none' there was a look of disbelief. The Nurse then Doctor were inquisitive about how I could be close to 60 and not taking any pills and appear to be in good health!

Energy healing is definitely not new, to the contrary it is ancient knowledge and practice. We lost our way by giving our healing power away to someone other than ourselves. We now have complete autonomous faith and hope in a person that has been trained to write prescriptions to 'mask' whatever is wrong with us. Most American Doctors do not claim to write prescriptions to **heal** you of your disorder. Simply to relieve you of the symptoms that you complain of having.

I have had numerous opportunities to use my Reiki knowledge to help others. It is especially satisfying when it is used to help an elder.

In December of 2013 I travelled to the West Coast to visit my family. My mother had gotten extremely ill from taking some pills her doctor of over twenty years had prescribed for her to take. She has given all of her health power over to this doctor. As she explained her experiences, my heart was in pain. How could this doctor carelessly prescribe something which could cause danger to my mother? I was highly upset, to say the least.

What compounded this matter was the fact the same doctor placed her in the hospital because her heartbeat was racing. My reply to him was she was fine the last she came to him and the only difference was she consumed the pills he had given her. Nonetheless, hospital bound she was because the family was concerned he had said the magic words 'the heartbeat' was racing.

This whole experience is forever etched in my memory, as a shaking my head in disbelief, as how the senior citizens are treated, or in this case mistreated. While in the hospital, when there was an absence of any visitors many of these patients were ignored while they **screamed** for help or assistance. On some occasions the nurse would go in and give them a pill and they would soon become dead quiet. I remember my mother's roommate told the nurse she could not take the pills she had for her. The Nurse asked her, my mother's roommate, if she were a doctor. That was so rude! What happened after the nurse insisted she take the pills were a spasmodic, trembling elder with reactions to the pills that she had told the nurse she was allergic to! When the hospital doctor responded to this patient, he confirmed that she should not have been given those pills. The nurse was reprimanded by the doctor.

So my mother who needed to believe in her decision to accept what her longtime doctor was telling her, was beginning to waiver and wonder. It appeared this team of hospital doctors were determined to perform a surgery, any surgery, on my mother. First it was her thyroid, next the gall bladder and then back to the thyroid.

I asked the thyroid specialist how many gall stones were needed to mandate the complete removal of a person's body organ? The response was, **it only takes 1!** I have personally done stone removals on my own body for nearly ten years and knew a person is capable of passing stones without surgery. The specialist was upset and appeared angry with me for having some knowledge of the function and/or removal of stones. He huffed at us, 'then she will have to sign a waiver that states she refuses the operation.' Hey that was the least of our worries.

Here is the magical solution. Later that evening once my mother fell asleep, I place my hands over her gall bladder and performed Reiki. This was not my first time yet I chose to do it while she was asleep. I wanted no interference at all. I said a prayer of invocation of

God, angels, ancestors and all guides who would help to be there with me. As my hands remained slightly resting on the area surrounding her gall bladder, I felt the stones moving along the artery in her body. It felt like a trickling of something small, like small rocks inside a tube.

Without question Energy Healing is an absolute must to improve and increase the quality of health and wellbeing for all of us but especially our elders. I cringe to think what could have happened had I not been there, the one who had knowledge on stones in the body and a Reiki practitioner. Regardless of the number of years we are alive here on Mother Earth, our existence should be one of peace and harmony with all living things. We should not suffer nor depend solely on pills to live.

Energy Healers are needed. Energy Healers will help save the lives of our elders. Energy Healers can enlist the help of our younger generation to create more active healers.

Will you help? Are you interested in becoming an Energy Healer? Would you like to fellowship with other Energy Healers to learn and ask questions?

CHAPTER 3

WHY – RESEARCH

SCIENTIFIC DATA – PLANT BASED NUTRITION

WHY RAW IS BETTER?

WHY? – THE RESEARCH

"Synergy – People have more energy when they eat well."

T. Colin Campbell, The China Study.

Dr. T. Colin Campbell, the author of a rather controversial book The China Study has come under some harsh criticism. His work in The China Study is sometimes critiqued on the grounds that it didn't prove that we shouldn't consume animal products; therefore, there's not enough evidence to follow a whole foods plant-based diet. However I disagree.

The work done in The China Study and over 350 scientific articles written by Dr. Campbell are impressive and holds merit on the grounds of the number of people included in the research (65,000 adults) and the amount of unbiased effort that was involved. The themes of the diverse human conditions and the lifestyles offer the world community a glimpse into the real mechanisms of our eating habits and its effect on our health. The data collected was from 65 counties across China where 376 variables were compared. We are aware of the disparities in health among the different economic groups of people. We know that money cannot save a person from suffering or contracting a dis-ease. However, considering the facts presented in this study it provides helpful information into means and ways to circumvent many dis-eases we face as a humanity. Upon completion of research more than 8,000 statistically significant associations between lifestyle, diet and disease variables were identified.

The sheer numbers that were researched is huge. Understanding the adoption of the Western world eating habits, we can often find cultures who were healthy at one time declining once they take on the habits of the Western civilization. I would offer this study as means to begin a conversation with your loved ones. What harm would it do, especially when America is fast losing the health game? Our natural, un-sprayed plant based foods are necessary for optimal longevity.

The work was completed with the help and assistance of expert Researchers from various Countries. It would seem unlikely that any type of cohesion took place. We must open our minds to look at new and different methodologies, if we are to change the direction of our health, especially for the sake of our children and their children's children.

There are thousands of research studies and reports that have been conducted on the benefits of eating a natural Whole Food Plant Based Diet (WFPBD). The inquisitive minds date back to the 1880's, when perhaps the research began. It is possible that it started even before the 1880's. Maybe the eating in the Garden by Adam and Eve that is depicted in the Holy Bible is the beginning of the truth that eating fruits and vegetables are the designed way to eat. The story does not include any animals that were consumed. Early humans ate fresh food from the Garden!

Nonetheless our technical advances have humanity eating all sorts of stuff these days. We ate animals, we eat items created in a laboratory that are GEO/GMO for means they are by no means a creation of Mother Earth. GEO/GMO stands for Genetically Engineered Organisms and Genetically Modified Organisms. The thought that these are called organisms sends a chill up my spine. The spinal cord functions primarily in the transmission of neural signals between the brain and the rest of the body but also contains neural circuits that can independently control numerous reflexes and central pattern generators. And Organism is defined by Merriam-Webster as: a complex structure of interdependent and subordinate elements whose relations and properties are largely determined by their function in the whole. In the creation of these organisms many times un-natural mixings or pairing occur. We cannot be absolutely sure of what is mixed together to create this new item that has been allowed to be called a food item.

If the ingredients were as harmless as the corporations that produce these items claim, why is billions of dollars spent by them to keep it secret and away from the general public's knowledge? Why should we trust people that do not trust us enough to give us the ingredients that included in what they are selling in stores? If not for anything other than the deceit of these corporations will I not support the items they create. Furthermore how is it possible to obtain a trademark, a patent on food?? The answer is that it is not wholly food, it has added ingredients that allows them to obtain a paten. That simply makes me sick to the stomach! Yet we eat it blindly, without thought to what we are ingesting or giving to our children to consume.

Many think they have no choice in the matter. These items are always cheaper and easier to find. The items last a long time on the store shelf and then on the shelf at your house. Ever wonder how long these things have been around? I have people who tell me that they bought some bread, forgot about it. Went on a month long vacation, only to return home to bread sitting on the table that is NOT MOLDED!! What harm that possibly cause to your body temple? How long is it staying in your system before being eliminated? Is it being eliminated? Many of the ingredients are not tested for human consumption before it is placed on the market for sell and use by you, the unsuspecting consumer.

So many of our animals are being abused, slaughtered without seeing the light of day ever, given growth hormones to rush them to the slaughter houses faster. What can this possibly do tour bodies? Are we then subjected to the same growth rate as the animals that we then eat? Is this why girls in American mature so much faster than girls in other Countries? What health consequences are we to experience when the effects of eating this type of diet is detected? Will the next generation be doomed to birth defects and illnesses that the medical professionals cannot cure? Will lifespans be shortened due to the damage caused by these un-natural ingredients? What is the question we should be asking, not only of ourselves but more importantly of the corporations that are being allowed to alter what we consume as food!!

Some of our children do not even know what 'real' food looks like. They think juice that comes in a bottle that is clear is real. Many have never been exposed to someone juicing real fruit or veggies to make 'real' juice. As far as this is concerned many adults may be lacking in knowledge with this also. How many understand that it is possible to cook your own meal without using a microwave oven or pop a covered container into the oven to get a meal? How many know having someone whom you do not know prepare the energy to fuel your body, your food, is not a good thing? How many even care? Yet Americans have the largest rates of obesity and other health problems in the world! And as Countries mimic or copy the Western style of eating their dis-ease rates go up accordingly. Is this what one would call a Fool's Paradise??

Medical Researchers have been perplexed about the role that medicines or pharmaceuticals play in the restoration of health. Medical professionals knew at one time in history, doctors were only compensated as their patients remained in good health. When the person became ill the doctor was no longer doing their job. How much of this medical system have changed? Is what we have now a 'sick-care' system, what happened to the notion that we should be WELL AND NOT SICK?? Why has the norm, the expectation changed? Why do we inherently assume that at a certain age we should have a certain ailment? Or that we need to begin taking supplements and pills at a particular age?

The fact there are many of Centenarians, individuals who live past 100 years of age that live a normal active productive life. I believe many more humans are capable of reaching this threshold as we accept we do have some control over our longevity. How we think and relate to others is a major component of living long years. I once served as a caregiver to a woman who lived until she was 103+. She always told me to do not worry about the small things in life, to count my blessings and be happy. I hear her words of wisdom all the time. She was jovial, did not entertain foolishness by anyone and knew how to avoid senseless acts of intolerance. She was kind and gentle and loved to sing. She had an active and alert mind. I loved me some Ruth Allen. I was one of her 'girls'!!

She had a fall at the facility where she resided and she suffered a broken bone in her leg. This made her immobile, she laid there in that hospital bed for days. This was so not her style of living. She was flat on her back. She did undergo rehabilitation but not too aggressive. Maybe the staff felt she had outlived the strength needed to regain her health and live additional days here on earth. It just seemed she sort of lost her will. I remember the last time visiting with her. She was not alert. I song a little, prayed a lot and kissed her on her forehead. I said goodbye and felt this was not the same as before when

I departed. I am blessed to have shared so much of this fabulous woman's life with her. Aunt Ruth remained a vital part of her community by years beyond what we think people should live. But Aunt Ruth served as my example of longevity. She was a few months short of being 104! What an honor to know and Love this woman of excellence!

So the biggest WHY is – do you believe you have the right to long life and if not why not? What I do know that is mandatory is your preparation for older aging. (Notice I did not say Old Age?) Without thought or planning, living beyond what the statisticians say is a normal lifetime may be a little daunting. Can you accept that even if you do not wish to be around longer than the number of years you determine, you can still live a healthier existence? The quality of your life is determined by you and the way you choose to eat and think.

Choose wisely. Live longer. Enjoy a higher quality of life. Have fun. Dance the night away. To your health!!

To sum this up, a quote from Dr. Campbell, The China Study, *"The entire system – government, science, medicine, industry and media – promotes profits over health, technology over food and confusion over clarity."*

SCIENTIFIC DATA

In studying it became apparently clear that information and knowledge is being kept in the secret chambers of the medical profession and not made available to the average person. The research data is in the Medical Journals, Medical Libraries, etc. Many of the statistics were new and unfamiliar to me. Yet the fact remains it is there and can be found with a little digging.

http://plantbasedresearch.org/ -

Welcome to plantbasedresearch.org, an online narrative review of peer-reviewed, scientific research papers and educational resources that are relevant to plant-based nutrition. Links to the abstract are included with every article, and links to the free full articles are included when possible! A narrative review is a collection of research papers supporting a particular theory - this website is by no means an exhaustive directory of all research on nutrition and disease but presents the growing body of evidence supporting the theory that whole food, plant-based diets offer the best chance for avoiding chronic disease, and in some cases, reversing it.

Here are just a few of the articles:

1. **Ethiopian pre-school children consuming a predominantly unrefined plant-based diet have low prevalence of iron-deficiency anemia.**
2. **Effects of Vegetarian Diets on Blood Lipids: A Systematic Review and Meta-Analysis of Randomized Controlled Trials.**
3. **Vegetarian, vegan diets and multiple health outcomes: a systematic review with meta-analysis of observational studies.**
4. **The moderate essential amino acid restriction entailed by low-protein vegan diets may promote vascular health by stimulating FGF21 secretion.**

Stanford Medicine Preventive Center -

http://nutrition.stanford.edu/projects/plant_based.html

We conducted a study designed to determine whether a plant-based diet consistent with the 2000 AHA dietary guidelines would be more effective in lowering blood cholesterol than the previously recommended low-fat, low-cholesterol diet. We randomly assigned 125 participants with moderately elevated cholesterol to eat either a plant-based diet, low in saturated fat and cholesterol but also rich in fiber, nutrients and phytochemicals, or a convenience foods-based diet with the same level of total and saturated fat and cholesterol.

After 4 weeks, (after only 4 weeks) the participants eating the plant-based diet, rich in nutrients and phytochemicals, reduced their total and LDL cholesterol significantly more than the participants consuming a standard low-fat diet. To learn more about the details of the study, read the Abstract published in the Journal Annals of Internal Medicine.

American Journal of Clinical Nutrition:

http://ajcn.nutrition.org/content/78/3/544S.full

Abstract

Evidence from prospective cohort studies indicates that a high consumption of plant-based foods such as fruit and vegetables, nuts, and whole grains is associated with a significantly lower risk of coronary artery disease and stroke. The protective effects of these foods are probably mediated through multiple beneficial nutrients contained in these foods, including mono- and polyunsaturated fatty acids, n-3 fatty acids, antioxidant vitamins, minerals, phytochemicals, fiber, and plant protein. In dietary practice, healthy plant-based diets do not necessarily have to be low in fat. Instead, these diets should include unsaturated fats as the predominant form of dietary fat (eq, fats from natural liquid vegetable oils and nuts), whole grains as the main form of carbohydrate, an abundance of fruit and vegetables, and adequate n-3 fatty acids. Such diets, which also have many other health benefits, deserve more emphasis in dietary recommendations to prevent chronic diseases.

By Frank B Hu

Dr. James McDougall

http://www.forksoverknives.com/science-says-about-diet-and-cancer/

A low-fat, plant-based diet* has been shown to positively affect survival in cancers of the:

Breast

Colon

Prostate

Skin: Melanoma

A truly therapeutic diet, like the McDougall Diet, is 7% fat with no meat, poultry, fish, eggs, dairy, or vegetable oils. Meaningful research in the future should use the best treatments available rather than compromise the patients' health with "prudent diets."

This enlightened dietary approach focuses on strengthening the human body and its magnificent abilities to heal and stay healthy; while, at the same time, removing cancer-causing and -promoting elements from the patients' diets. Even diseases, which seem as far removed from food as pre-cancerous actinic keratosis of the skin and lung (smoking) cancer are benefited with a healthy low-fat diet. The McDougall Diet supports phenomenal recoveries in many ways.

On February 13, 2015, the American Cancer Society published their recommendations that cancer survivors should follow "prudent diets," plant-based diets that are high in fruits, vegetables and unrefined grains while at the same time being low in red and processed meats, refined grains, and sugars. Its report states, "These diets are contrasted to 'Western' diets,' which have the opposite pattern and are heavy in meats, sweets, other processed foods, and dietary fat." They also recommend weight loss and exercise in order to prolong survival for people with cancer.

American Institute for Cancer Research (AICR)

http://www.aicr.org/about/advocacy/the-china-study.html?referrer=https://www.google.com/

AICR's Recommendations for Cancer Prevention are based on our expert report and the Continuous Update Project – independent, systematic reviews of the global scientific literature supplemented by the analysis and judgments of an expert panel.

Those judgments became AICR's 10 Recommendations for Cancer Prevention. Five of these relate specifically to the shape of a cancer-protective diet:

- **Limit consumption of energy-dense foods (like fast foods) and avoid sugary drinks.** (This recommendation aims to help us stay at a healthy weight.)
- **Eat mostly foods of plant origin, like vegetables, fruits, whole grains and legumes.**
- **Limit how much red meat you eat and avoid processed meat.** (Eat less than 18 ounces (cooked) of beef, pork or lamb per week; avoid smoked, cured or salted meats).
- **Limit alcoholic drinks.** If you drink, limit to no more than two drinks a day for men and one drink a day for women.
- **Limit consumption of salt.**

These five Recommendations add up to a diet than can contain some, little or no animal products. **AICR's review of the evidence does not show an additional benefit from following a completely vegan diet.** In our review, poultry and fish are not linked to increased risk for any specific cancers.

AICR does not make any specific recommendations about dairy products. Our Expert Report and Continuous Update Project indicate that there is strong evidence that milk and calcium are linked to a decreased risk of colorectal cancer. However, our reviews also indicate that there is 'limited but suggestive' evidence that dairy products and diets high in calcium increase the risk of prostate cancer. This is an active area of investigation as researchers design studies to better understand these findings, so stay tuned.

An easy way to picture AICR's dietary advice: at every meal, fill at least 2/3 of your plate with plant foods and 1/3 or less with animal foods.

Doctor T. Colin Campbell

http://nutritionstudies.org/t/plant-based-diet/

Written by Thomas Campbell, MD

Preventing and Treating Erectile Dysfunction (ED)

Think of the manliest scenes in American culture: downing meat, eggs, and protein to 'bulk up' or sitting in front of a TV with chicken wings and pizza, watching the game, or grilling a steak while pounding beers, . These 'manly' activities may actually be the exact opposite of what your penis needs to be functional over time.

Instead, to prevent and treat erectile dysfunction, step away from the steak, hot dogs, and chicken wings and try some beans, fruit, and vegetables and get off your butt and get your heart rate up regularly. When we look beyond pop culture, and the dangerous stereotypes of masculinity, science tells us that those are actually the factors that make for the best sexual function over your lifetime.

See the full article at above link.

Hippocrates Health Institute

http://hippocratesinst.org/

For more than forty years, Ann Wigmore, founder of the renowned Hippocrates Health Institute and internationally acclaimed holistic health educator, taught that what we eat profoundly affects our health. She was among the first to note that our modern diet of "convenience food" was the prime cause of illness and obesity, and she offered a positive alternative.

Developed over a twenty-year period at the Hippocrates Health Institute, one of the nation's first and finest holistic health centers, the Hippocrates Diet allows the body to correct its problems naturally and at its own pace. Through a diet of fresh fruits, vegetables, grains, nuts, and super nutritious foods such as sprouts and wheatgrass juice, all of which are prepared without cooking, the body is able to restore its internal balance—and its capacity to maintain a healthy weight, fight disease, and heal itself.

# # #

Brenda Cobb
http://www.livingfoodsinstitute.com

Brenda Cobb, Founder and Director of Living Foods Institute, overcame breast and cervical cancer without the use of chemotherapy, radiation or surgery by following the simple principles that are taught in her Healthy Lifestyle Programs today. She eliminated all allergies, migraine and sinus headaches, acid reflux, indigestion, heartburn, rheumatoid arthritis, age and liver spots, and gray hair. Her eyesight even improved! She is completely healthy and looks and feels many years younger than her actual age. Brenda now devotes her life to educating and helping others.

Brenda was awarded an Honorary Cultural Doctorate in Therapeutic Philosophy from the World University in September 2003 for her work in helping people heal from diseases that the medical community thought were terminal, incurable and hopeless.
Living Foods Institute is located in Atlanta, Georgia.

# # #

I have pulled different articles to address a variety of health issues. You can do your own research if this is insufficient for you. There are tons of information and research on the topic of Whole Foods Plant Based Diet.

WHY RAW IS BETTER

When following a raw diet, cooked is any food that is cooked above 115 degrees, food retains the natural nutrients that are inherent and readily accessible for our quality of healthy living when it is raw.

Brenda's Story
http://www.livingfoodsinstitute.com/about_meetBrenda.php

This is not your typical before and after story, this is the testimony of one woman's all natural total healing from cancer and how she turned her personal health crisis into a gift for the world. In 1999 **Brenda Cobb** was diagnosed with breast and cervical cancer. Her doctor said she most likely would be dead in 6 months to a year if she didn't do surgery, chemotherapy and radiation. She didn't do anything the doctor recommended and she healed completely all the natural way!

Brenda's reason for not wanting to follow her doctor's recommendations was because many personal family members with breast, cervical, uterine and ovarian cancers had done chemotherapy, radiation and surgery only to have cancers return with a vengeance and to lose their lives. Brenda knew that poisoning the body in the name of healing did not work and she was determined to find a different and natural way to support her body to do what it was created to do – heal itself.

How did she do it? Brenda nourished her body with all Organic, Vegan, Raw and Living Foods, detoxified and cleansed her colon, lymphatic system and blood; cleared out and healed emotional stuff she had buried inside, and in six months she was completely healed! Brenda used to be plagued with allergies, arthritis, depression, chronic fatigue, headaches and skin problems, but now that is all in the past. Today she is vibrantly healthy and radiant!

# # #

Ann Wigmore's Story –

http://hippocratesinst.org/ann-wigmore-founder

The story of Hippocrates Health Institute began in **1908**, when Ann Wigmore was born in Lithuania. To learn more about the factors of her youth that shaped her future, read her compelling biography, "Why Suffer?" At the age of 13, she sailed to the United States to reunite with her parents, who were already living in Massachusetts. She eventually married, had a daughter and lived a simple, humble life in Stoughton, a town about 10 miles south of Boston.

While Ann was raising her family, a Danish doctor by the name of Kristine Nolfi was diagnosed with breast cancer in **1940.** She refused established medical protocol and successfully treated herself with an exclusively raw food diet. When she regained her health, she opened a health center called Humlegaarden where she treated many patients with cancer and other diseases.

A decade or so after Dr. Nolfi had reversed her cancer, Ann, in poor health and suffering from colon cancer, began to incorporate the lessons she recalled learning as a child in Lithuania from her grandmother, the village doctor, who treated wounded soldiers with herbs during World War I. Using weeds and wheatgrass, she also healed her body and reversed the cancer. Witnessing the powerful healing properties of wheatgrass juice and other vitamin and enzyme-rich foods first-hand inspired her to spend the next 35 years of her life studying and educating others about natural healing and optimum nutrition.

# # #

David Servan-Schreiber, MD., PhD.

http://www.prevention.com/food/food-remedies/one-doctors-personal-food-cures-cancer

I was diagnosed with brain cancer about 16 years ago. I received chemotherapy and went into remission, but the cancer came back and I endured two surgeries and 13 months of chemotherapy. I asked my oncologist if I ought to change my diet to avoid another recurrence. His answer was perfectly stereotypical: "Eat what you like. It won't make much difference."
In my quest, I discovered that the list of cancer-fighting foods is actually quite long. Some foods block natural bodily processes such as inflammation that fuels cancer growth. Others force cancer cells to die through a process that specialists call apoptosis. Still other foods assist the body in detoxifying cancer-causing toxins or protecting against free radicals. But most of them attack the disease on a variety of fronts. And they do it every day, three times a day, without provoking any side effects. To avoid the disease, it's essential to take advantage of this natural protection, and nurture it.

I've learned that the anticancer diet is the exact opposite of the typical American meal: mostly colorful vegetables and legumes, plus unsaturated fats (olive, canola, or flaxseed oils), garlic, herbs, and spices. Meat and eggs are optional. Through extensive research, I devised a list of the most promising cancer fighters, along with recommendations on how to make the most of their potential. Include at least one, and preferably two, at every meal, to maximize your protection.

#

CHAPTER 4

FOOD

DETOX

WATER

URINE THERAPY

FOOD

FDA to Start Testing for Glyphosate in Food

The federal agency already tests for residues of many agricultural chemicals on food. Now it will include the widely used weed killer linked to cancer.

By Carey Gillam on **February 17, 2016**

Filed Under: Pesticides

The U.S. Food and Drug Administration (FDA), the nation's chief food safety regulator, plans to start testing certain foods for residues of the world's most widely used weed killer after the **World Health Organization's** cancer experts last year declared the chemical <u>a probable human carcinogen.</u>

The FDA's move comes amid growing public concern about the safety of the herbicide known as glyphosate, and comes after the U.S Government Accountability Office (GAO) rebuked the agency for failing to do such assessments and for not disclosing that short-coming to the public.

<u>*Private companies, academics, and consumer groups have recently launched their own testing and claim to have detected glyphosate residues in breast milk, honey, cereal, wheat flour, soy sauce, infant formula, and other substances.*</u>

FDA officials dubbed the issue "sensitive" and declined to provide details of the plans, but FDA spokeswoman Lauren Sucher said the agency was moving forward to test for glyphosate **<u>for the first time in the agency's history.</u>**

"The agency is now considering assignments for Fiscal Year 2016 to measure glyphosate in soybeans, corn, milk, and eggs, among other potential foods," she told Civil Eats. Soybeans and corn are common ingredients in an array of food products and genetically engineered (or GMO) varieties are commonly sprayed with glyphosate.

#

What a better way than to open this chapter with current news! Is it possible that the FDA has allowed this toxic chemical to be used throughout America on our crops and just now realize it is causing dangers to human lives? I find that astonishing and downright apprehensible. How can the governing body of Food and Drugs not know the dangers in the chemicals used to spray the very commodity it protects and governs??

We had seriously do a better job at regulating what we eat than to allow the policy makers to do it for us. This toxic chemical has been allowed free will in the spraying on our crops for years. Many responsible organizations and community focused groups have called for action well before now to no avail. The information has been called to the attention of the government officials for years now. Elections are held throughout the nation to mandate that these companies tell the consumers what are the ingredients and their effect on the human lives. Now that WHO is filing charges against Monsanto's Round-Up weed killer the FDA wants to now investigate?

In parts of our Nation, growers, farmers are paid NOT to grow on their land. Other farmers are being sued because the sprayed chemicals have contaminated their crops! Yes that is correct. If the manufacturers of this chemical can prove that a trace amount exist in the farmers' crops they can be sued for illegally using the substance of which they had no rights to use! The law is tilted against the honest, hardworking American farmer. The big companies and corporations have taken control and we are eating the spoils of such a calamity.

More of the article:

The FDA effort comes during an intense political debate over perceived risks of genetically modified crop technology to human health and the environment, and glyphosate residues on food is a key concern. Several states have moved to mandate labeling of foods made with GMOs, and one such measure in Vermont is set to take effect July 1. Many large food industry players and agribusiness interests are fighting mandatory labeling and seeking a federal bill that would block Vermont's law.

The FDA move to start testing was cheered by Michael Hansen, senior staff scientist at Consumers Union, though Hansen said the USDA must not continue to duck the issue. The USDA's annual pesticide data program (PDP), in operation since 1991, is considered the primary authoritative report on pesticide residues on food.

But critics say several studies have linked glyphosate to human health ailments, including non-Hodgkin lymphoma and kidney and liver problems, and because glyphosate is so pervasive in the environment, even trace amounts can be harmful due to extended exposure.

# # #

FOOD EMPOWERMENT PROJECT

http://www.foodispower.org/

FOOD IS POWER

Food Empowerment Project seeks to create a more just and sustainable world by recognizing the power of one's food choices. We encourage choices that reflect a more compassionate society by spotlighting the abuse of animals on farms, the depletion of natural resources, unfair working conditions for produce workers, the unavailability of healthy foods in communities of color and low-income areas, and the importance of not purchasing chocolate that comes from the worst forms of child labor.

Dietary Diseases

While the causes of coronary heart disease and diabetes may vary, scientific evidence from dietary studies has linked the consumption of animal products to these deadly ailments. Additional research has correlated consuming vegan foods (plant based) with a lower risk of heart disease, diabetes, and a whole host of other chronic and debilitating disorders. For some people, improving their diet can be as simple as deciding to eat healthier foods, but for others it can be much more challenging—especially if they have limited or no access to healthy foods like fresh produce and whole grains in the areas where they live.

More than one-third of US adults have some form of cardiovascular disease, which is the leading cause of death in the US, and 8.3 percent of the population suffers from type 2 diabetes. Adults with diabetes are also at high risk for cardiovascular disease, with 65 percent of diabetes sufferers dying from heart disease or stroke. Unhealthy dietary habits and a lack of physical activity play major roles in the development and progression of both heart disease and type 2 diabetes.

The diabetes death rate for African Americans is 40.5 per 100,000, an incidence that is more than double the diabetes rate for whites. One probable cause of this disparity is that communities of color are more likely to be located in food deserts, which are geographic areas where residents' access to affordable, healthy food options is restricted or nonexistent due to the absence of grocery stores within convenient traveling distance.

Eating for Health

The official position of the American Dietetic Association (ADA), the world's largest organization of food and nutrition professionals, is that healthy vegan and vegetarian diets "can help prevent and treat chronic diseases including heart disease, cancer, obesity and diabetes."

According to the ADA, "Vegetarian diets tend to be lower in saturated fat and cholesterol and have higher levels of dietary fiber, magnesium and potassium, vitamins C and E, folate, carotenoids, flavonoids and other phytochemicals. These nutritional differences may explain some of the health advantages of those following a varied, balanced vegetarian diet." The report also stated that plant-based diets are appropriate for people of all ages and activity levels, including pregnant and nursing mothers, infants, children, adolescents, and athletes

Food for Thought

However you slice the facts and figures, it is clear that coronary heart disease and diabetes stem from the same risk factors—eating animal products and processed foods, unhealthy weight gain, and lack of exercise. People can significantly reduce their risk factors for these and other diseases by making healthy lifestyle choices.

You may think that changing what you eat will be difficult because it can be tied to your moods, your health or your economic and social circumstances, and living in a food desert can make it even more challenging. However, what you eat can prevent or reduce your risk of dietary diseases and premature death, so choosing plant-based foods can truly be empowering, healing and even life-saving.

# # #

Food, what an odd topic of discussion. Especially when the conversation is centered on healthy eating. Many will turn a deaf ear rather than hear what is being discussed in regards to their current diet. Even if the food of choice is making us sick and obese, there are those who would choose to stay unhealthy instead of making a change in eating habits. Food is our lifeline. We will perish or prosper because of it. What will be your choice?

My sincere prayer is that you choose to take a serious look into your choices and determine you want to live a higher quality of life. It is not all doom and gloom with regards to aging. Nor is it only a few that can be spared with illness or swallowing a massive amount of pills just to survive. We each have the power to change our journey. We can have health abundantly. When we choose and make right decisions based upon the natural nature of life, we are in concert with Mother Earth. How Divine is that? To your Good Eating!!

DETOX

Detoxing is crucial for optimum health. There are thousands of toxins and chemicals we are exposed to every single day. Depending on your age that could translate to hundreds of thousands of hours and days of your exposure to these toxins which can harm the body. If this is your first time considering your health from a Wholistic standpoint you may truly be harboring a ton of toxins in your system.

When our body temples are cleaned they function more efficiently. Less need of pharmaceuticals to treat or correct any conditions or dis-ease you may be experiencing in your life. There are numerous methods to utilize to cleanse your body. Personally I do both a liver and colon cleanse regularly to maintain a healthier body. But keep in mind that there are many more suitable and viable cleanses on the market. Personally I prefer the ones that I make myself. Others prefer kits or herbs that are already mixed for their needs. It does not matter to me which you choose, as long as you do a body cleanse of the liver and colon. These are the first two organs used in your digestive system. It stands to reason that if these two are not functioning properly that your food is not being absorbed by your body to provide you with the optimum. The foods you are ingesting are only partially serving you and your health needs.

When the liver is clogged, food is not assimilated and passed through with ease. Food struggles to distribute its nutrients and minerals to your organs, tissues and cells. You are only receiving partial benefit from all the hard and dedicated work you are doing. This is my motivation to do these very inexpensive cleanses on a regular basis.

Oh and just a word of caution and advice. My first time out the gate in doing a cleanse it lasted for 40 days. I felt great only after the 3rd day. Friends that began with me did not make it to the 3rd day. However my energy soared after that crucial 3rd day. Here is the remarkable happening. I did colon cleanses faithfully every three months. It was not until the end of the second year that I released such foul odors from my body that I knew it had to be stuff that was stuck way deep inside my colon!! When I tell you the smell was awful. That would be an understatement. My personal experience confirms what I had been told for years, even though we have bowel movements on a regular daily basis we can still be constipated or old stuff can be clogged up in our intestines. Of course I did not believe this when it was originally told to me by a Naturopathic Practitioner.

Blogger Kristen Nagy says, "Toxic agents are everywhere in our world. The food we eat, the air we breathe, the household cleaners we spray, and the electronics we use on a daily basis… However, toxic free radicals are formed in the body too. Stress hormones, emotional disturbances, anxiety and negative emotions all create free radicals as well. Living without toxic buildup is virtually impossible, which is why our body has built in mechanisms to deal with toxic overload. Crying, sweating, urination and defecation are all natural protocols employed by the body to rid itself of toxins. Detoxification is so important because it can literally reverse the symptoms of illness and change your life. There are many different types of detoxification protocols and it is important to find one that works well for you. The liver, small intestine, kidneys, and colon are the major organs involved in the body's detoxification system. However, when employing any type of cleanse (like a juice cleanse, liver and gallbladder cleanse, elimination diet, heavy metal cleanse, etc.) it is important to first cleanse the kidneys and colon, as these two eliminative organs are responsible for carrying toxic waste out of the body."

<u>Simple Detox Methods:</u>

1 – 3 day juice fast (Monthly)
Use any of the following ingredients –

Apples	Bok Choy
Carrots	Cranberries
Cantaloupe	Papaya
Apricots	Leafy Greens
Red Grapes	Watermelon

# # #

1 – 10 day water fast (Monthly)
Start your month by cleansing the first few days. After a day or so you are full of energy and clear-thinking. No brain-fog nor mind chatter. Keeps you on track and focused.
4 Day Apple Cleanse – (Will aide with constipation also)

Eating apples serve as an excellent method to getting all the dietary fiber your body needs to promote colon health. On top of that apples are said to be rich in the water-soluble dietary fiber pectin that serves to jellify salts, sugars, and fat, nutrients that get stored away as fat, serving as an active fat blocker.

Apples also contain a dietary fiber called cellulose to help detoxify your body sending toxins out cleaning your system as well as stimulating your digestive tract effectively relieving constipation promoting healthy gut flora.

Amongst other things the apple diet is a well-known single food complete diet as well as a replacement diet used in substitution to normal healthy eating habits to quickly decrease your calorie intake while acting as a colon cleanse. All you have to do is eat nothing but apples for a 4 day period.

Daily Cleansing –

1. Upon waking in the morning, drink a Liter of clean water. This will cause you to have a bowel movement within 30 minutes or so. Be certain to use clean fresh water. Suggestion: either purchase alkaline water or make it yourself by adding lemon or lime to distilled water overnight. Or you can boil your water and allow it to sit overnight. The

boiling removes the toxins from the water. This is a very old, tried and true solution to buying bottled water. The water is amazingly tasty!

2. Make a tea of lemons and hot boiling water. This concoction is both alkalizing and detoxifying.

3. At bedtime, mix 2 tablespoons each of organic olive oil and fresh organic lemon juice. Shake well and drink. Lay on your right side for at least 20 minutes. This will help clean your liver overnight.

4. Liver Parasite cleanse – ½ cup organic coconut shreds, ½ cup organic coconut oil, make into balls the size of ½ tablespoons. Eat 4 to 6 at a time.

5. Diatomaceous Earth destroys cancerous energy form the body and parasites from the stomach and liver.

6. Do organic coffee enemas.

7. Detox Salad
    a. Arugula or mixed greens
    b. Avocado
    c. Cucumber
    d. Cilantro
    e. Dulse – Seaweed flakes
    f. Dressing
        i. 1 Tablespoon Organic Virgin Olive Oil
        ii. 1 Teaspoon ACV – Apple Cider Vinegar
        iii. Place in a glass jar and shake well before pouring over salad

This is a repost of one of my Health Blogs: Keeping Your Insides Cleaned

Researchers have found most average everyday Americans are constipated, not able to have a bowel movement at least 2-3 times per day, but junk like raw sewage is built up on the walls of the intestines preventing a complete release of the body's waste. If you have less than 2-3 bowel movements per day you are experiencing health issues, i.e. gout, headaches, acid reflux, etc.

COLON CLEANSING

I recommend The Master Cleanse by Stanley Burroughs, because I know of two vibrant young men where this cleanse saved their lives! These are two virile, strong, otherwise healthy young thirty something year old young men!

One had been on the cleanse for forty days, competing with me to see how long we could go before stopping. He had an attack at the conclusion which was his appendix 'exploding' on his insides. The Surgeon advised him he would had died had it not been for the fact his system was clean and clear of all food particles. The appendix contains poisons and attaches itself to food found in the stomach when it erupts. Per the doctor the only thing that saved his life was the fact he had been on the cleanse as long as he had.

The other young man was rushed to emergency, he had high blood pressure, high cholesterol, high everything that should not had been. After two weeks on the cleanse and exercising daily, his return visit to the doctor revealed a weight reduction of thirty pounds and all vital signs completely within a normal range! There is no need to be placed on any medicines.

The little book, **The Master Cleanser** by Stanley Burroughs cost less than $7.00. You also save money while on the cleanse, as you clean out your system. You do not eat any food and you will not get hungry! It is beneficial to increasing your overall health. Your energy SOARS after the first 2 or 3 days. Depending on the amount of toxins and waste in your body, you may experience headaches, facial blemishes or fatigue. This is due to the toxins being cleaned from your system. This is all discussed in the book.

Once the toxins are released, optimum health is yours!

Personally, I do a colon cleanse every 3 to 4 months, more often if I choose to eat out a lot. I also do a liver cleanse once a year. There can be stones preventing your liver from functioning as it is designed. It is your first line of defense in the digestion of everything you eat. My first experience I passed more than 300 stones from my liver and I had been regularly cleansing my colon for about 3 years! More on liver cleanse in an upcoming issue.

I recently learned of another method for interior cleansing and it is Apple Cider Vinegar. Dr. Bragg has several books on health issues and one specifically on the benefits and detailed instructions on the Apple Cider Vinegar Miracle Health System. He explains how to control weight and banish obesity, uses as an internal and external health tonic, learn these powerful health qualities for a longer, healthier, youthful life. My brother followed this system with outstanding results with clearing out an infection his medical regimen could not.

THE MASTER CLEANSE by STANLEY BURROUGHS

THE MASTER CLEANSE DIET

The Master Cleanse Lemonade

The lemonade is prepared by mixing the ingredients in this free recipe:

- **2 tablespoons freshly squeezed lemon juice.** Burroughs recommends organic lemons, fresh, not bottled juice. Limes may be substituted. Lemon zest and pulp may be added, making sure that the lemons are organic and not artificially colored or treated with pesticides.
- **2 tablespoons of maple syrup.** This must be pure maple syrup, not pancake syrup. Burroughs recommends the darker Grade B, which has more color and nutrients than Grade A, which is also acceptable. He goes into aspects of maple syrup production that would be difficult for the average person to investigate, such as whether formaldehyde or plastic tubing is used (not recommended by Burroughs).
- **1/10 teaspoon cayenne pepper.** Burroughs insists that cayenne chili pepper be used, but permits ramping up from a lesser amount if the taste needs getting used to.
- **Water.** Burroughs recommends a 10-ounce glass of medium hot water, but also allows cold water to be used. Some have interpreted "10-ounce glass" to mean 8 ounces of actual water. Since Burroughs also allows plain water to be drunk during the fast in addition to the lemonade, this doesn't seem important.

An alternative to the lemonade endorsed by Burroughs substitutes 10 ounces of fresh sugarcane juice for the lemon juice and water. But few people are going to have access to fresh, organic sugar cane juice. Some people who can not stomach the maple syrup taste have substituted an equal number of calories of powdered sugarcane or organic cane sugar, available from some health food stores (one user described it as tasting like pond scum, worse than the maple syrup).

Things to Avoid at All Costs

Burroughs strongly counsels against the use of **honey** in the lemonade or the consumption at any time of honey, which he describes as **predigested bee vomit,** popular only among "gullible health foodists."

Burroughs also cautions against taking any kind of **supplements** or **vitamin pills** or using illicit drugs. Although Glickman wisely recommends against going off any **prescription medications** without your doctor's approval, it's unclear what Burroughs' opinion was on this point. He reprints without comment an endorsement from a follower who relates how he quit his medications for blood pressure, nerves, and lack of energy during his fast. And Burroughs was generally against traditional medicine in general, discouraging a leukemia patient from getting a bone marrow transplant. And an alternative version of the Master Cleanse for diabetics described in the book recommends that the diabetic phase out insulin during the diet. In another context in the book Burroughs rails against "the unnatural action of drugs and antibiotics," saying they store "poisons in the body." But we're with Glickman on this one.

You shouldn't smoke or drink **alcohol, coffee, tea, cola**, but the good news is that your cravings for them will completely disappear, according to Burroughs. Burroughs allows the consumption of extra **plain water** and of **mint tea**. No other food or drink should be consumed at all, say both Burroughs and Glickman.

The Colon Blaster

There are two preparations needed to induce colon cleansing.

- **Laxative herb tea.** Although Burroughs is quite specific about types and amounts of lemons and maple syrup, on the subject of laxative herb teas he simply suggests without further elaboration that you should buy any good brand offered by your health food store.
- **Internal salt water bathing solution.** Dissolve two teaspoons of un-iodized sea salt in a quart of lukewarm water.

The laxative herb tea and the salt water are the one-two punch that will keep your colon in full-time Old Faithful mode during the diet, cleansing it clean as a whistle.

During the Diet

To begin the diet you need to choose the minimum number of days that you are going to attempt, steel yourself for what is to come, and follow the following daily routine.

Day 0 (the day before beginning the diet):

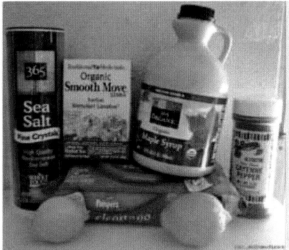

Purchase lemons, maple syrup, cayenne pepper, laxative herbal tea, and sea salt in sufficient quantities to last the duration of your cleanse.

Purchase a large supply of toilet paper and Tucks® brand witch hazel wipes or **Pre-moistened toilet wipes are excellent.** If you share your bathroom with others, agree on a unique emergency code phrase like "It's coming," "Dr. Livingston, I presume," or "Elvis is leaving the building" to alert other members of your household that you need them to vacate the bathroom quickly; also, consider purchasing a supply of adult diapers.

The night before beginning the diet, drink some laxative herbal tea, and retire for the evening.

Days 1 through 10 (and Beyond):

- In the morning before drinking any lemonade, drink a quart of salt water (remain near a toilet).
- During the day drink 6 to 12 glasses of the Master Cleanse lemonade concoction. The lower number of 6 glasses is recommended for those seeking weight loss. The higher number is fine for those interested mostly in detoxification.
- In the evening drink some herbal laxative tea.
- You may experience dizziness, vomiting, joint pain, and weakness. This is due to the toxins being released from your system. After several days many Master Cleanse dieters report entering a state of bliss that is probably the result of the continuing elimination of toxins.

Note: Over the years since Stanley Burroughs' death variations of the original Master Cleanse described here have developed, and attempts at clarifying ambiguous points have been made. Peter Glickman's book, as well as this popular internet based book by Raylen Sterling, deal with some of these modifications to the Master Cleanse orthodoxy.

Post Diet: Breaking the Fast

When are you through with the diet? Either when you reach the number of days that you planned, or alternately, when your tongue goes from "coated and fuzzy" to a clear pink color.

<u>Burroughs outlines a gentle approach for coming off the diet without upsetting your digestive system excessively.</u> Although Burroughs recommends that you become a practicing raw foodist vegetarian after the diet to avoid recontamination with toxic dead animal flesh, he does provide an alternative transition plan for omnivores.

Vegetarian Transition Process

- **Days 1 and 2:** Drink several 8-ounce glasses of orange juice, sipping slowly, diluting it if there is digestive distress.
- **Day 3:** Drink orange juice in the morning, eat raw fruit for lunch, and eat fruit or raw salad for dinner.
- **Day 4:** You may return to your normal diet.

Omnivore Transition Process

- **Day 1:** Drink several 8-ounce glasses of orange juice, sipping slowly, diluting it if there is digestive distress.
- **Day 2:** Drink orange juice during the morning and afternoon. For dinner prepare a homemade vegetable soup (recipe below). Mostly sip the broth, and do not eat much of the vegetables.
- **Day 3:** Drink orange juice in the morning, have leftover vegetable soup for lunch with 4 rye crackers (no regular crackers or bread), and eat fresh raw vegetables, salad, and fruit for dinner. *Do not yet eat meat, fish, eggs, bread, pastries or drink tea, coffee, or milk.*
- **Day 4 and beyond:** You may return to your normal diet, but Burroughs recommends continuing to drink the lemonade concoction at breakfast on a permanent basis. And he really wants you to go vegetarian, if at all possible.

Master Cleanse Recipe: The Omnivore Vegetarian Soup

Ingredients:

- 2 varieties of beans, 1/2 cup each (kidney beans, lentils, pinto beans, or other)
- 1 medium potato, half-inch cubes
- 1 stalk celery, sliced
- 1 carrot, sliced
- 1 small bunch turnip greens, spinach, mustard greens or other green
- 1 onion, diced
- 3 medium tomatoes
- 1 green pepper, diced
- 1 zucchini, sliced
- 1/2 cup brown rice
- Other vegetables as desired
- *No meat*
- 1 teaspoon cumin
- 1 teaspoon dry oregano
- 1 teaspoon curry powder

- 1/8 teaspoon cayenne pepper
- 1 teaspoon salt
- vegetarian soup powder or cube (optional)

Preparation:

Combine ingredients with 4 cups water, bring to a simmer, cook 20 minutes or until potatoes and beans are tender, adding water along the way if necessary.

Protein and the Master Cleanse

The Master Cleanse provides several hundred calories of carbohydrate per day in the form of lemon and maple sugar, and Burroughs' recommended vegetarian diet excludes "toxic dead animal flesh." What about protein? In the case of protein, Burroughs says that there is no need to worry: protein is simply nitrogen, oxygen, hydrogen, and carbon. The air contains all these elements. Simple by breathing "we are able to assimilate and build the nitrogen also into our bodies as protein ... by natural bacteria action...." But just to be on the safe side, Burroughs also recommends eating nuts and seeds after the Master Cleanse.

Master Cleanse Alternatives

There are other cleanses out there, and many dieters spend time looking into the Master Cleanse vs. water fast, Master Cleanse vs. juice fast, and Master Cleanse vs. Colonics.

Quotations from Stanley Burroughs

On germs, viruses and epidemics:

"In recent times it has been believed that these many diseases are contagious and that germs have spread them....

"Disease, old age, and death are the result of accumulated poisons and congestion throughout the entire body. These toxins become crystallized and hardened, settling around the joints, in the muscles, and throughout the billions of cells all through the body ... Lumps and growths are formed all over the body as storage spots for unusable and accumulated waste products ... These growths and lumps appear to us as forms of fungi....

"When we stop feeding this fungi and cleanse our system ... they dissolve or break up and pass from the body.... Germs and viruses do not and cannot cause any of our diseases ... Germs and viruses are in the body to help break down waste material and can do no harm to healthy tissues....

"Basically, all of our diseases are created by ourselves because we have never taken the time to discover the true foods meant for man's use.

"Since germs do not cause our disorders, there must be another logical reason for the triggering of an epidemic. This is a matter of simple 'vibration.' The better the physical and mental condition a person is in, the higher becomes his vibration, but as he steadily becomes clogged with more and more waste matter, his vibration goes constantly downward...."

On his imprisonment for practicing medicine without a license:
"After dedicating a goodly share of my past life in perfecting and simplifying a system of healing that is completely free from error and side effects, at a very low cost, I was forced to overcome many difficult obstacles that often threatened to stop me, but I persisted in spite of the medical and legal attacks. *I was told in each case I was doing too much good,* and to keep me from giving the help that solved their health problems I was sent to prison so I couldn't help anyone any more. But ... many of the guards, nurses and even doctors [in prison] came to me for help that no other system could [offer]. In prison I was not competing with their medical rackets, but on the outside I hurt their con games, If my system was made legal, the medical system would be of no further need."

Stanley Burroughs: 1903-1991

RECIPE FOR LIVER CLEANSE

Ingredients

- 4 tablespoons Epsom salts
- one-half cup of olive oil - the light olive oil is easier to drink
- 1 large or 2 small fresh pink grapefruit (enough to squeeze 2/3 to ¾ cup of juice)
- Ornithine, 4 to 8 capsules, to help you sleep. People have done the cleanse without Ornithine

Steps:

- Choose a day like Saturday for the cleanse, since you will be able to rest the next day. Take no medicines, vitamins or pills that you can do without; they can prevent success. Eat a no-fat breakfast and lunch such as:
  - a cooked cereal with fruit
  - fruit juice
  - bread and preserves or honey (no butter or milk)
  - baked potato or other vegetables with salt only.

  This allows the bile to build up and develop pressure in the liver. Higher pressure pushes out more stones.

- 2:00 PM. Do not eat or drink anything but water after 2 o'clock. If you break this rule you could feel quite ill later. Get your Epsom salts ready. Mix 4 tbs. in 3 cups of water and pour this into a jar. This makes four servings, ¾ cup each. Set the jar in the refrigerator to get ice cold (this is for convenience and taste only).

- 6:00 PM. Drink one serving (3/4 cup) of the ice cold Epsom salts. (Recommended: Drink the Epsom salt solution through a straw to get the drink to the back of your mouth and avoid most of the taste. A little maple syrup afterwards sweetens the aftertaste of the salts.)

- 8:00 PM. Repeat.

- 9:45 PM. Pour ½ cup olive oil into pint jar. Add ¾ cup squeezed grapefruit juice. Shake vigorously.

- 10:00 PM. Drink this mixture taking 4 to 8 Ornithine capsules (not mandatory but helps one sleep). Lie down immediately on your back with head high on your pillow. Keep perfectly still for at least 20 minutes. Go to sleep
(Recommended: A warm hot water bottle placed on your upper abdomen and slightly to the right helps your liver to relax.)

- Upon Awakening - After 6 AM. Take third dose of Epsom salts.

- 2 Hours Later. Take fourth dose of Epsom salts.

- 2 Hours Later. You may eat starting with juice and fruit. Later eat light.

LIVER CLEANSE INFORMATION

Cleansing the liver of gallstones dramatically improves digestion, which is the basis of your whole health. You can expect your allergies to disappear, too, more with each cleanse you do! Incredibly, it also eliminates shoulder, upper arm, and upper back pain. You have more energy and increased sense of well-being.

It is the job of the liver to make bile, 1 to 1 ½ quarts in a day! The liver is full of tubes (biliary tubing) that deliver the bile to one large tube (the common bile duct). The gallbladder is attached to the common bile duct and acts as a storage reservoir. Eating fat or protein triggers the gallbladder to squeeze itself empty after about twenty minutes, and the stored bile finishes its trip down the common bile duct to the intestine.

For many persons, including children, the biliary tubing is choked with gallstones. Some develop allergies or hives but some have no symptoms. When the gallbladder is scanned or X-rayed nothing is seen. Typically, they are not in the gallbladder. Not only that, most are too small and not calcified, a prerequisite for visibility on X-ray. There are over half a dozen varieties of gallstones, most of which have cholesterol crystals in them. They can be black, red, white, green or tan colored. The green ones get their color from being coated with bile.

At the very center of each stone is found a clump of bacteria, according to scientists, suggesting a dead bit of parasite might have started the stone forming.

As the stones grow and become more numerous the back pressure on the liver causes it to make less bile. Imagine the situation if your garden hose had marbles in it. Much less water would flow, which in turn would decrease the ability of the hose to squirt out the marbles. With gallstones, much less cholesterol leaves the body, and cholesterol levels may rise. Gallstones, being porous, can pick up all the bacteria, cysts, viruses and parasites that are passing through the liver. In this way "nests" of infection are formed, forever supplying the body with fresh bacteria. No stomach infection such as ulcers or intestinal bloating can be cured permanently without removing these gallstones from the liver.

Cleanse your liver twice a year.

How well did you do?

Expect diarrhea in the morning following the cleanse steps. Use a flashlight to look for gallstones in the toilet with the bowel movement. Look for the green kind since this is proof that they are genuine gallstones, not food residue. Only bile from the liver is pea green. The bowel movement sinks but gallstones float because of the cholesterol inside. Count them all roughly, whether tan or green. You will need to total 2000 stones before the liver is clean enough to rid you of allergies or bursitis or upper back pains permanently. The first cleanse may rid you of them for a few days, but as the stones from the rear travel forward, they give you the same symptoms again. You may repeat cleanses at two-week intervals.

A Gallstone flush is the second most important thing someone can do in order to cure "incurable" and degenerative diseases. "This procedure contradicts many modern medical viewpoints. Gallstones are thought to be formed in the gallbladder, not the liver. They are thought to be few, not thousands. They are not linked to pains other than gallbladder attacks. It is easy to understand why this thought: by the time you have acute pain attacks, some stones in the gallbladder are big enough and sufficiently calcified to see on X-ray, and have caused inflammation there. When the gallbladder is removed the acute attacks are gone, but the bursitis and other pains and digestive problems remain." People who have had their gallbladder removed surgically still get plenty of green, biliary stones. Dr. Ted Morter D.C. says the removal of the gallbladder increases chances of osteoporosis.

Dr. H.H. Worrell did extensive work in this field and was the creator of this Liver Cleanse. He was treating me for Crohns Disease and towards the end of my treatment with him was when he finalized the steps and was able to share this with me. Dr. Worrell died shortly after making this discovery of how the liver must be totally cleaned and functioning to be able to overcome any digestive disorders. Or simply to get the body operating perfectly.

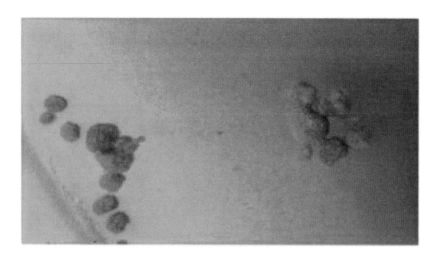

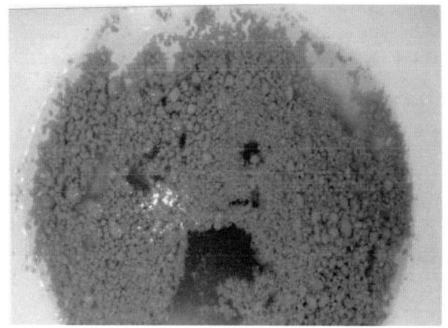

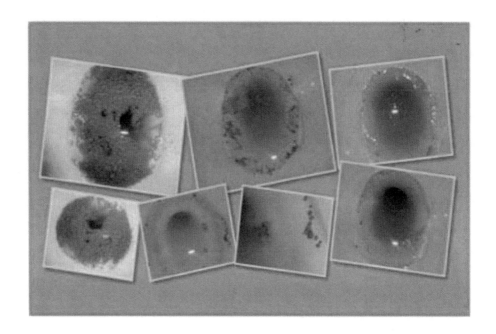

These are actual pictures from a liver cleanse that I did in 2013.
Note the sizes and number of stones that I passed!

TWO ADDITIONAL DETOXIFICATION METHODS

BENEFITS OF A COFFEE ENEMA

For many years I suffered from **systemic candida**, and didn't get results with conventional medicine. In fact, I became more unwell thanks to endless rounds of synthetic drugs that were being prescribed to me.

I decided to take my health into my own hands, and began my holistic journey of getting back to health.

Along the way I discovered the powerful benefits of coffee enemas in helping rid the body of Candida. Candida loves to hang out with the liver, and that by doing coffee enema's regularly, they will help flush out the candida along with nasty toxins from the liver.

Enemas have been around since the dawn of time and have even been recorded in biblical scripts. They are making a comeback as people are starting to see the health benefits of including enemas into their daily routines.

Coffee enemas are powerful detoxifiers, due to some amazing compounds within the coffee that stimulate the liver to produce Glutathione S transferase, a chemical which is known to be the master detoxifier in our bodies.

Glutathione S transferase binds to toxins and the toxins are then released out of the body along with coffee.

Detoxifying our bodies on a regular basis is more important than ever due to the increasing amount of toxins our bodies need to deal with every day, from home to office, man made products, food, water, the air we breathe, and our busy stressful lifestyles.

Here are 10 Reasons on Why You Should Try A Coffee Enema:

1. Reduces levels of toxicity by up to 600%.
2. Cleans and heals the colon, improving peristalsis.
3. Increases energy levels, improves mental clarity and mood.
4. Helps with **depression**, bad moods, and sluggishness.
5. Helps eliminate parasites and candida.
6. Improves digestion, bile flow, eases bloating.
7. Detoxifies the liver and helps repair the liver.
8. Can help heal chronic health conditions (along with following a mainly raw plant based diet).

9. Helps ease "die-off" or detox reactions during periods of fasting or juice fasting, cleansing or healing.
10. Used regularly in the Gerson Institute treatment protocol for healing cancer patients naturally

Even if you're sensitive to caffeine, it won't affect you taking your coffee this way. (Definitely do not attempt to use decaf coffee though, you won't get the benefits.) By taking it orally, the coffee goes through your digestive system and stomach acids, which nullify any benefits you'd get if you took your coffee via the portal vein to the liver!

Buy some premium ground ORGANIC coffee beans and keep them in the freezer until you need to use the coffee.

Ideally do your coffee enema after a bowel movement, so you can retain the coffee for longer. So mornings are best for most people. If you are constipated, do the enema anyway, this will get things moving nicely!

Grab a saucepan and put 2 tablespoons of organic coffee in the saucepan. Add 3 cups of **FILTERED** water to the pot.

Bring to a boil and let simmer for 15 minutes. Remove from heat after 15 minutes and let it cool. When it's body temperature strain through a nut milk bag into a clean glass pouring jar.

Head to the bathroom with your strained coffee and set up a space and something comfortable for you to lie down on. Hint: Be near a toilet and use an old towel as you sometimes may get slight coffee leakage. Grab a pillow and some reading material as you will be here for approximately 12 to 15 minutes.

Now assemble your enema kit. It must have a tube and nozzle attached to the bucket or bag. Make sure it's at least 1 meter above ground.

There will an attachment near the nozzle that allows you to stop or start the flow of coffee once you have poured it into the bag or bucket. Ensure this is in the off position before pouring the coffee into the bag!

Once the coffee is in the bag or bucket hold tube and nozzle over sink or shower plug and turn it on and allow the coffee to run through the tube until there are no air bubbles. Stop the flow again once this is done.

Grab some coconut oil and apply to the nozzle for ease of insertion. Lie down on your towel on your right hand side with your knees drawn up.

Insert the nozzle till it's about 1 inch inside the rectum. Turn on the flow of coffee slowly until the bag or bucket is emptied.

Now you can either remain lying on your **right side** or lie on your back with your feet up above head level or feet resting against a wall above head level. You can even do some yogi moves like a shoulder stand or a half plough type position, this helps get the coffee moving round nicely, you may also hear some funny squirting noises from your tummy, this is a good sign and an indication of the bile being stimulated for release.

Try to retain the enema for 12 to 15 minutes. You may feel some strong urges to go to the toilet, especially the first few times you try this. Try to hold on for as long as you can, quite often the sensations pass. As you do them more regularly you will be able to retain for longer. 15 minutes max is all you need.

When you are ready to release head to the toilet and let it go.

You should feel a lot lighter in body and mind by now!

Coffee enemas are very safe and are <u>sometimes taken up to 6 times a day in chronically ill patients</u>. If you are healing, on a detox program, or cleansing, I recommend daily enemas. For maintenance, I recommend weekly enemas.

If you are wishing to remove candida and pathogens, <u>try 3 back-to-back,</u> and continue to do them on a regular basis.

OIL PULLING – ORAL HEALTH
Author: Unknown

Oil pulling is an ancient Ayurvedic practice dating back thousands of years. When it harnesses the antimicrobial power of coconut oil, you have one very powerful tool! The high lauric content of coconut oil makes it a strong inhibitor of a wide range of pathogenic organisms, from viruses to bacteria to protozoa. Researchers in Ireland found that coconut oil treated with enzymes, in a process similar to digestion, strongly inhibits Streptococcus bacteria, which are common oral residents that can lead to plaque buildup, cavities, and gum disease.

Oil pulling can lessen your toxic load by pulling out pathogens and preventing their spread to other areas of your body. When done correctly, oil pulling has a significant cleansing, detoxifying and healing effect. Oil pullers have reported rapid relief from systemic health problems such as arthritis, diabetes and heart disease. Sesame oil is traditionally recommended, but it has a relatively high concentration of omega-6 oils. Therefore, I believe coconut oil is far superior, and to me it tastes better. But from a mechanical and biophysical perspective, both oils likely work.

Oil pulling is simple. Basically, it involves rinsing your mouth with about a tablespoon of coconut oil, much like you would using a mouthwash. The oil is "worked" around your mouth by pushing, pulling, and drawing it through your teeth for a period of about 15 minutes. If you are obsessive like me, you can go for 30-45 minutes. This process allows the oil to neutralize and "pull out" bacteria, viruses, fungi and other debris. After working the oil around for 15 minutes, spit it out and rinse your mouth with water. Do NOT swallow the oil as it's loaded with bacteria and toxins. Naturopathic physician and coconut oil expert Bruce Fife compares the benefits of oil pulling to changing the oil in your car:

"It acts much like the oil you put in your car engine. The oil picks up dirt and grime. When you drain the oil, it pulls out the dirt and grime with it, leaving the engine relatively clean. Consequently, the engine runs smoother and lasts longer. Likewise, when we expel harmful substances from our bodies our health is improved and we run smoother and last longer."

Your Diet Is Key to Reducing Chronic Inflammation

The running thread linking a wide variety of common health problems, including cancer, is *chronic inflammation* in your body – regardless of whether it originates in your mouth or not. Clearly, addressing your oral health is an important step, but it really all **starts** with your diet.

Your diet can make or break your teeth, as it were, and has a profound effect on your overall level of inflammation. Therefore, to optimize your health and prevent many of the diseases listed above, you'll want to evaluate your lifestyle to ensure you're doing everything you can to *prevent chronic inflammation* from occurring. To reduce or prevent inflammation in your body, you'll want to avoid the following dietary culprits:

- Sugar/fructose and grains

- Oxidized cholesterol (cholesterol that has gone rancid, such as that from overcooked, scrambled eggs)

- Foods cooked at high temperatures

- Trans fats

Beyond that, brushing with baking soda and using oil pulling can help address the bacterial balance in your mouth. The most important factor, however, is to regularly reseed your gut with beneficial bacteria, i.e. probiotics. Fermented vegetables and other traditionally fermented foods are an ideal source, but if you don't eat fermented foods, then a high-quality probiotic is certainly recommended.

Four Strategies for Improving Your Oral Health

The latest research uncovering the connection between the microorganisms in your mouth and cancer make it extraordinarily clear that oral hygiene is a necessary Prerequisite if you want to be healthy. Major problems can result from the overgrowth of opportunistic oral pathogens, including oropharyngeal cancers, colorectal cancer, and if you're an expectant mother, even the tragedy of stillbirth. In addition to avoiding fluoride and mercury fillings, my top four recommendations for optimizing your oral health are as follows:

1. Consume a traditional diet: fresh fruits and vegetables, grass-pastured meats, poultry, eggs, and dairy; nuts and seeds; minimal consumption of sugar and processed food
2. Add in some naturally fermented foods, such as sauerkraut, pickles, kimchee, yogurt, kefir
3. Proper brushing, flossing, and cleaning between teeth with a small brush.
4. Oil pulling

A traditional diet will help balance both your oral and gastrointestinal flora, but it may not be enough to guarantee perfect oral health. I've struggled with plaque for years, and it wasn't until I added fermented foods and oil pulling that I began to make progress with the problem. The addition of fermented foods decreased my plaque by 50 percent and made it much softer, and the oil pulling has improved it further.

Poor Oral Health Is a Risk Factor for Oropharyngeal Cancers

The human papillomavirus (HPV), some strains of which are associated with cervical cancer if left untreated for long periods of time, has similarly been linked to vaginal, vulvar, penile, anal, and oropharyngeal cancers (cancers of the throat, tonsils, and base of tongue).

Hence the ridiculous recommendation to vaccinate boys with the notorious HPV vaccine, Gardasil, which is riddled with dangerous side effects and other problems. A new study published in the journal *Cancer Prevention Research* reports:

"Poor oral health, which includes dental problems and gum disease, is an independent risk factor for oral HPV infection, and by extension, could also contribute to oral cancers."

In this study, participants with poor oral health had a 56 percent higher rate of HPV infection than those with healthy mouths. Centers for Disease Control and Prevention states that about 60 percent of oropharyngeal cancers are related to HPV, but according to the latest study, it could be as high as 80 percent.

The researchers speculate that good oral hygiene could help prevent HPV infection, thereby lowing your risk for oropharyngeal and other cancers. Human papillomavirus is actually a group of more than 100 viruses. Of those 100, about 40 are sexually transmitted, and 15 of those are the types most often associated with cervical cancers and genital warts.

It is important to note that more than 90 percent of women infected with HPV **clear the infection naturally within two years**, at which point their cervical cells return to normal. It is only when the HPV virus lingers for many years (that is, *becomes chronic*) that abnormal cervical cells could turn into cancer.

This is why regularly scheduled PAP smears prevent cervical cancer deaths far more effectively than the HPV vaccine ever will, because they allow a sufficient amount of time to find and treat any cervical abnormalities.

Viruses Cause 15 to 20 Percent of All Cancers

It is interesting to note that HPV isn't the only virus linked to cancer—in fact, it is estimated that 15 to 20 percent of all cancers are caused by viruses! Many viruses trigger cancer by suppressing your immune system and/or altering your genes. The following viruses are known to play a major role in certain types of cancer:

- EBV (Epstein-Barr virus) increases your risk for nasopharyngeal cancer, certain lymphomas and stomach cancer

- Hepatitis B and C are linked to liver cancer

- HIV is associated with invasive cervical cancer, lymphoma, lung cancer, liver cancer, anal cancer, oropharyngeal cancer, skin cancer and Kaposi's sarcoma; Herpes virus 8 is also thought to be involved with almost all cases of Kaposi's sarcoma

Three New Studies Prove Oral Bacteria Can Cause Colorectal Cancer

There is one bacterium that has been causing a great deal of trouble with people's health: *Fusobacterium nucleatum*, a spindle-shaped anaerobic bacterium commonly found in dental plaque. *F. nucleatum* is abundant in your mouth and able to coaggregate with other species. Three recent studies have linked *F. nucleatum* with serious health problems:

1. Case Western Reserve University researchers found that some malignant colorectal tumors are caused by *F. nucleatum*
2. Harvard researchers also established a link between *F. nucleatum* and the initiation of colorectal tumors
3. A study in *Journal of Obstetrics and Gynecology* found that oral *F. nucleatum* can lead to intrauterine infection and even stillbirth

The first two studies establish *an actual causal link* between this bacteria and colorectal cancer. The bacteria trigger inflammation and also activate the cancer growth genes and the signals required for angiogenesis to occur (a tumor's blood supply). Normally, *F. nucleatum* is not prevalent in your gut, but if your microbial balance is off—which can happen in your mouth, as well as in your gut—then it's able to invade and colonize. *F. nucleatum* has been found in gut mucosal biopsies that show inflammation and in biopsies of colorectal tumors.

The third study discusses an unusual case of a mother losing her baby to stillbirth due to an intrauterine infection, *directly resulting from gingivitis*. The bacteria moved from her mouth to her uterus because her immune system was weakened by a respiratory infection. Other studies have shown these bacteria to cause stillbirths in mice, but this was the first documented human case.

All of these studies unequivocally show that bacterial imbalances and dysbiosis can contribute to inflammation in your body and activate cancer genes. Therefore, the bacteria in your mouth deserve as much care and attention as the ones in your gut. Not surprisingly, they're interrelated, and as you improve your gut flora, the flora in your mouth improves accordingly. I experienced this myself. When I started consuming fermented vegetables, it only took a few months before I was able to reduce the frequency of my visits to my dental hygienist for a persistent plaque problem.

Another Danger: A Mouthful of Mercury

Besides oral hygiene, which I'll be discussing shortly, there are two other dental-related concerns you may need to address: mercury amalgams and fluoride. The average American has eight mercury amalgams (fillings), falsely described as "silver" fillings. This misleading label has been purposely used to keep you in the dark about the exact composition of the fillings, which are actually about 50 percent mercury. Mercury is a toxic heavy metal that can poison your brain, central nervous system and kidneys. Children and fetuses, whose brains are still developing, are most at risk—but anyone can be adversely impacted.

Mercury is such a potent toxin that just one drop in a lake would poison the lake to the extent that the Environmental Protection Agency (EPA) would ban fishing in it. Yet, they claim that carrying around a mouthful of mercury fillings has no harmful effects. If you have mercury amalgams, it would be advisable to consult a holistic, mercury-free dentist.

Steer Clear of Fluoride in Any Form

If you are using fluoridated toothpaste, you may want to consider tossing it out and replacing it with a safe one. In the mornings, you could use toothpaste containing calcium and phosphate salts, or even hydroxyapatite, which can help re-mineralize your teeth. Baking soda will help promote beneficial bacteria in your mouth by neutralizing the acid that pathogenic bacteria thrive in. I use an oral irrigator with baking soda twice a day and follow with coconut oil pulling for 20 minutes.

Fluoride is of little or no benefit to your teeth and poses serious health risks, including immune dysfunction, endocrine disruption, increased risk of fractures, arthritis, infertility, and many more.

Toothpaste isn't the only source of fluoride—it is present in growing numbers of non-organic foods from pesticide residue (including iceberg lettuce). And fluoride continues to be added to many municipal water supplies in the United States. Water fluoridation has come under increasing scrutiny as health concerns, lack of efficacy in preventing tooth decay and ethical issues of administering chemicals via the water supply have surfaced.

For more information on fluoride, please watch the presentation by Michael Connett, an attorney with the Fluoride Action Network.

AND LASTLY.... WATER AS A DETOXIFIER

The Health Benefits of Water

Functions
Water losses
Water vs. other beverages
How much is enough?
Adding water to your routine

The human body is a water machine, designed primarily to run on water and minerals. Every life giving and healing process that happens inside our body... happens with water. In just the last decade medical science has begun to focus more on the tremendous healing ability our body has and how much that ability depends on water. Our body instinctively knows how and strives to sustain youthful longevity, and in its every effort... water is the key. The human body is made up of over 70% water. Our blood is more than 80%, our brain ... over 75%, and the human liver is an amazing 96% water!

Our energy level is greatly affected by the amount of water we drink. It has been medically proven that just a 5% drop in body fluids will cause a 25% to 30% loss of energy in the average person... a 15% drop in body fluids causing death! Water is what our liver uses to metabolize fat into useable energy. It is estimated that over 80% of our population suffers energy loss due to minor dehydration.

Functions

Water is a fundamental part of our lives. It is easy to forget how completely we depend on it. Human survival is dependent on water -- has been ranked by experts as second only to oxygen as essential for life. The average adult body is 55 to 75% water. 2/3 of your body weight is water (40 to 50 quarts). A human embryo is more than 80% water. A newborn baby is 74% water. Everyday your body must replace 2 1/2 quarts of water. The water you drink literally becomes you! Since such a large percentage of our bodies is water, water must obviously figure heavily in how our bodies function. We need lots of fresh water to stay healthy.

Water is the medium for various enzymatic & chemical reactions in the body. It moves nutrients, hormones, antibodies, & oxygen through the blood stream & lymphatic system. The proteins & enzymes of the body function more efficiently in solutions of lower viscosity. Water is the solvent of the body & it regulates all functions, including the activity of everything it dissolves & circulates.

Water helps regulate our body temperature through perspiration, which dissipates excess heat & cools our bodies.

We even need water to breathe! As we take in oxygen & excrete CO_2, our lungs must be moistened by water. We lose about 1 to 2 pints of water each day just exhaling.

Asthma is frequently relieved when water intake is increased. Histamine plays a key role in regulating the way the body uses & distributes water & helps control the body's defense mechanisms. In asthmatics, histamine level increases with dehydration. Our defense for the body is to close down the airways.

The kidneys remove wastes such as uric acid, urea & lactic acid, all of which must be dissolved in water. When there isn't sufficient water, those wastes are not effectively removed, which may result in damage to the kidneys.

Water lubricates our joints. The cartilage tissues found at the ends of long bones & between the vertebrae of the spine hold a lot of water, which serves as a lubricant during the movement of the joint. When the cartilage is will hydrated, the two opposing surfaces glide freely, & friction damage is minimal. If the cartilage is dehydrated, the rate of "abrasive" damage is increased, resulting in joint deterioration & increased pain.

The actively growing blood cells in the bone marrow take priority over the cartilage for the available water that goes through the bone structure.

Rheumatoid joint pain frequently decreases with increased water intake & flexing exercises to bring more circulation to the joints.

75% of the upper body weight is supported by the water volume that is stored in the spinal disc core. 25% is supported by the fibrous materials around the disc. The spinal joints are dependent on different hydraulic properties of water which is stored in the disc core. Back pain is frequently alleviated with hydration.

Brain tissue is 85% water. Although the brain is only 1/50th of the body weight, it uses 1/20th of the blood supply. With dehydration, the level of energy generation in the brain is decreased. Depression & chronic fatigue syndrome are frequently results of dehydration.

Migraine headaches may be an indicator of critical body temperature regulation at times of "heat stress." Dehydration plays a major role in bringing on migraines. Dehydration causes stress & stress causes further dehydration.

Water losses

Adults lose nearly 6 pints (12 cups) of water every day. We lose 1/2 cup to 1 cup a day from the soles of our feet. Another 2 to 4 cups is lost from breathing. Perspiration accounts for another 2 cups. Another 3 pints (6 cups) are lost in urine.

When the body is dehydrated, a form of rationing & distribution goes into play to ration the available water. Since the body has no reserve system, it operates a priority distribution system for the amount that has been made available by intake.

The body's signals of dehydration are frequently joint pain, stomach pain & ulcers, back pain, low energy, mental confusion & disorientation. Numerous disease symptoms respond to increased water intake.

If you're not drinking sufficient water, your body starts retaining water to compensate for this shortage. To eliminate fluid retention, drink more water, not less. If you don't drink enough water to maintain your body's fluid balance, you can impair every aspect of your body's physiological function.

The "dry mouth" signal is the last outward sign of extreme dehydration. As our bodies try to adjust to being deprived of water, our thirst mechanism becomes disabled. The only time we receive the "dry mouth" signal is as the last outward sign of extreme dehydration. In addition, the thirst sensation gradually decreases with age. The result is increasing dehydration. As we start to give our bodies more water, the thirst mechanism begins to work again, but doesn't become fully apparent until our bodies are fully hydrated. When we are getting sufficient water, we're often thirsty.

Water vs. other beverages...

There is a difference between drinking pure water & beverages that contain water. Fruit juice, soft drinks, coffee, etc., may contain substances that are not healthy, & actually contradict some of the positive effects of the added water. Caffeinated beverages stimulate the adrenal glands and act as diuretics, robbing your body of necessary water. Soft drinks contain phosphorus which can lead to depletion of bone calcium. Soda contains sodium. Fruit juices contain a lot of sugar & stimulate the pancreas. These drinks may tax the body more than they cleanse it. A 12 ounce can of regular soda contains the equivalent of 9 teaspoons of sugar and loads of empty calories.

Other beverages also contain dehydrating agents. They may actually reduce the water reserves in the body! Drinking other beverages to the exclusion of water also causes you to lose your taste for water. This is particularly true with children as they become dependent on Sodas & juices.

How much is enough?

A non-active person needs a half ounce of water per pound of body weight per day. That is ten 8 ounce glasses a day if your weight is 160 pounds. For every 25 pounds you exceed your ideal weight, increase it by one 8 ounce glass.

An active, athletic person needs 2/3 ounce per pound which is 13-14 8 ounce glasses a day if you're 160 pounds. The more you exercise the more water you need. Spread out your water intake throughout the day. Do not drink more than 4 glasses within any given hour. After a few weeks your bladder calms down & you will urinate less frequently, but in larger amounts.

Adding water to your routine

Here are a few tips for adding more water to your life:

Keep a supply of water containers full in the fridge. That way, water is always on hand as an alternative to other less healthful drinks and conveniently available when you're on the go.

Upon arriving at the office, fill up a big jug of water at the tap. You'll get plenty of water to drink throughout your workday.

Caffeinated beverages act as diuretics and increase fluid loss, so they don't count toward your daily hydration needs. Try substituting water for your second cup of coffee or that mid- afternoon soda.

Don't wait for your body to signal it's thirsty. By that time, you're already starting to be dehydrated.

URINE THERAPY

What You Don't Know Can Hurt You

Every one of us has a right to know that our bodies produce an invaluable source of nourishment and healing that we can utilize to heal ourselves and to maintain our lives and our health in both everyday circumstances and in emergencies and life-threatening situations. Two news articles from the past that recently came across my desk vividly illustrate the absolutely tragic consequences of the public's lack of information and our completely unfounded misconceptions regarding our bodies' own perfect medicine: *Tom Brokaw, NBC Nightly News, October 16, 1992*: "In Egypt, rescue workers found a 37-year-old man alive in earthquake rubble. He survived almost 82 hours by drinking his own urine. His wife, daughter and mother would not and they died." *Associated Press, July, 1985*: I don't think there's any question that these women and the child would not have died had they simply been aware of the truth that not only would their own urine not harm them, but would, in fact, have provided a power-packed combination of liquid nutrients and critical immune factors that would have sustained them in good health until help arrived.

The Medical Proof

For almost the entire course of the 20th century, unknown to the public, doctors and medical researchers have been proving in both laboratory and clinical testing that our own urine is an enormous source of vital nutrients, vitamins, hormones, enzymes and critical antibodies that cannot be duplicated or derived from any other source. They use urine for healing cancer, heart disease, allergies, auto-immune diseases, diabetes, asthma, infertility, infections, wounds and on and on — yet we're taught that urine is a toxic waste product. This discrepancy between the medical truth and the public information regarding urine is ludicrous and, as the news releases you've just read demonstrate, can mean the difference between life and death to you and to your loved ones. When I contracted a crippling, incurable disease early in life, I used every available conventional medical and alternative healing method over the course of many years without success. When an acquaintance suggested I try "urine therapy" I thought she'd lost her mind, but with no options left, I swallowed my prejudice and decided to give it a go. To my own (and everyone else's) amazement, my healing was so rapid and so profound with urine therapy that no question remained in my mind that someone in the medical community had to know more than they were telling about this incredible body substance. And as a matter of fact, they did know more – a lot more. After many months of haunting university libraries, scanning countless microfiche files and poring over piles of medical journals, I had amassed a small mountain of astounding research studies, findings and files on the use of urine in medicine and healing. I discovered, among numerous other things, that urine, far from being a toxic body waste, was actually a purified derivative of the blood made by the kidneys which contains, not body wastes, but rather an incredible array of critically important nutrients, enzymes, hormones, natural antibodies and immune defense agents. At the end of it all, as I sat tiredly in my chair eyeing the stacks of research papers covering my desk, I realized that the medical community had pulled off one of the biggest hoodwinks in history. Take for instance the doctor who reported that "urine acts as an excellent and safe natural vaccine and has been shown to cure a wide variety of disorders including hepatitis, whooping-cough, asthma, hay fever, hives, migraines, intestinal dysfunctions, etc. It is completely safe and causes no side effects." (J. Plesch, M.D., The Medical Press, 1947); or the oncologist who reported that "a patient with intractable ovarian cancer was treated with Human Urine Derivative and is now completely well and enjoying the rest of her life." (Dr. M. Soeda, University of Tokyo, 1968). These remarkable findings were published in medical journals – but did you ever hear about them? And what about the immunologist who, after extensive clinical and laboratory research stated: "It was rapidly appreciated that undiluted urine administered orally was therapeutically effective for Immune Therapy and was initiated when it became obvious that an allergic condition had become uncontrollable." (Dr C.W. Wilson, 1983, Law Hospital, Scotland) Or the Harvard medical researchers who discovered that active "antibodies to cholera, typhoid, diphtheria, pneumonia, polio, leptospira and salmonella have been found in the un-concentrated urine of infected individuals." (Lerner, Remington & Finland, Harvard Medical School, 1962) What about the Scandinavian researcher who, in 1951, conclusively proved that human urine can completely destroy tuberculosis? It's a deadly disease, and is now resistant to antibiotics. Isn't it time someone told us that our own urine is medically proven to be anti-tubercle? Then there's the research into wounds and burns using urea (the primary solid component of urine). As only one research study among many reported: "In America, urea has been used for the treatment of various infected wounds and it has been found to be extremely efficient...even the deepest wound can be treated effectively.... Urea treatment has been successful where other treatments have failed. For external staph infections we found urea preferable to any other dressing...there are no contra-indications to its use." (Dr. L. Muldavis, 1938, Royal Free Hospital, London) Now these medical reports are only a few of the more than 50 research studies I compiled and published in the book Your Own Perfect Medicine, but they certainly give an indication of the importance of what we've never been told about urine by the medical community. As far back as 1954, the Journal of the American Medical Association (July issue) reported that "More scientific papers have probably been published on urine than on any other organic compound." Another publication revealed that "more than 1,000 technical and scientific papers, related only to low molecular weight substances in urine, appeared in medical and scientific literature in one single year." All this fuss about a substance that we're told is nothing more than a body waste? I think one of the most interesting pieces of information on urine I came across was the fact that the amniotic fluid that surrounds human infants in the womb is primarily urine. Actually, the infant "breathes in" urine-filled amniotic fluid continually, and without this fluid, the lungs don't develop. Doctors also believe that the softness of baby skin and the ability of in-utero infants to heal quickly without scarring after pre-birth surgery is due to the therapeutic properties of the urine-filled amniotic fluid. Reports on the extraordinary external benefits of urine abound as well. Medical studies relate remarkable cases of stubborn or "incurable" chronic, severe eczema that miraculously disappear with urine therapy. Because urine is both anti-viral and anti-bacterial, it's ideal for treating cuts, wounds and abrasions of all kinds. Acne, rashes, athlete's foot and fungal skin problems respond dramatically to urine soaks and compresses as well. (You'll find complete instructions for using urine therapy internally and externally in Your Own Perfect Medicine.) For home use or emergency treatment care for wounds, poisonous bites or stings, and even broken bones, urine is an incomparable, proven natural healing agent that provides instantaneous therapeutic benefits under any circumstances. For years, people have said to me, "Well, I have heard of people surviving by ingesting their own urine, but I thought it was just a myth." Myth it isn't. Medical fact it is. As Dr. John R. Herman remarked in his article which appeared in the New York State Journal of Medicine in June, 1980: "Auto-uropathy (urine therapy) did flourish in many parts of the world and continues to flourish today ... there is unknown to most of us, a wide usage of uropathy and a great volume of knowledge available showing the multitudinous advantages of this modality. Actually, the listed constituents of human urine can be carefully checked and no items not found in human diet are found in it. Percentages differ, but urinary constituents are valuable to human metabolism."

Your Body's Own Super-Nutrition Therapy

In 1975, one of the founders of Miles Laboratories, Dr. A.H. Free, published his book Urinalysis in Clinical Laboratory Practice, in which he remarked that not only is urine a sterile body compound (purer than distilled water), but that "it is now recognized that urine contains thousands of compounds, and as new, more sensitive analytical tools evolve, it is quite certain that new constituents of urine will be recognized." Among the urine constituents mentioned in Dr. Free's revealing treatise is a list of nutrients that will knock your socks off. As Dr. Free comments, the ingredients listed below are only a few critical nutrients found in urine.

- Alanine, total ..... 38 mg/day
- Arginine, total ..... 32 mg/day
- Ascorbic acid ..... 30 mg/day
- Allantoin ..... 12 mg/day
- Amino acids, total ..... 2.1 g/day
- Bicarbonate ..... 140 mg/day
- Biotin ..... 35 mg/day

- Calcium .... 23 mg/day
- Creatinine .... 1.4 mg/day
- Cystine .... 120 mg/day
- Dopamine .... 0.40 mg/day
- Epinephrine .... 0.01 mg/day
- Folic acid .... 4 mg/day
- Glucose .... 100 mg/day
- Glutamic acid .... 308 mg/day
- Glycine .... 455 mg/day
- Inositol .... 14 mg/day
- Iodine .... 0.25 mg/day
- Iron .... 0.5 mg/day
- Lysine, total .... 56 mg/day
- Magnesium .... 100 mg/day
- Manganese .... 0.5 mg/day
- Methionine, total .... 10 mg/day
- Nitrogen, total .... 15 g/day
- Ornithine .... 10 mg/day
- Pantothenic acid .... 3 mg/day
- Phenylalanine .... 21 mg/day
- Phosphorus, organic .... 9 mg/day
- Potassium .... 2.5 mg/day
- Proteins, total .... 5 mg/day
- Riboflavin .... 0.9 mg/day
- Tryptophan, total .... 28 mg/day
- Tyrosine, total .... 50 mg/day
- Urea .... 24.5 mg/day
- Vitamin B6 .... 100 mg/day
- Vitamin B12 .... 0.03 mg/day
- Zinc .... 1.4 mg/day

As you read over this extraordinary list of nutritional elements, you can begin to understand why the stories you may have heard of people surviving on their own urine are true. But what about other elements in urine that you've heard about?

Clearing Up the Misconceptions

If you asked a person on the street what uric acid is, he or she would invariably answer that it's a toxic body waste. Not so, say medical researchers at the University of California at Berkeley who in 1982 reported they had discovered that "uric acid destroys body-damaging, cancer-causing free radicals and is considered to be one of the physiological factors that enable human beings to live so much longer than other mammals." But what about urea? Urea is in urine and isn't that the toxic stuff that causes uremic poisoning? Actually, medical researchers discovered many decades ago that urea, far from being a toxic body waste, is an incredibly versatile, far-reaching and effective medicinal agent. In numerous medical studies, it was shown that urea is one of the most potent non-toxic virucidal agents ever discovered. In one particular study, the rabies and polio virus [sic] were killed so quickly and efficiently by concentrated urea, that even the laconic researchers themselves were surprised: "Urea is such a relatively inactive substance and certainly not a protoplasmic poison such as are most virucidal agents, that it is in a way surprising that rabies and poliomyelitis are killed so easily by urea solutions" (McKay & Schroeder, Society of Experimental Biology, 1936). In reality, Urea is an FDA-approved medicinal agent that doctors and researchers utilize in an amazing variety of therapeutic modalities. Because of its remarkable and comprehensive anti-neoplastic (anti-tumor) properties, it's presently being used in anti-cancer drugs and is extensively studied for use in cancer treatments. The urea compound drug, glicazide, is used successfully by the medical establishment in treating both insulin-dependent and non-insulin-dependent diabetics. As a natural diuretic, urea is unparalleled, and is a proven and accepted treatment in cases of edema or swelling such as excess cerebral and spinal pressure, glaucoma, epilepsy, meningitis, even premenstrual edema and many other disorders in which excess fluid is a problem. As one American neurosurgeon reported regarding a patient who nearly died from complications following brain surgery: "Urea was administered intravenously as an emergency measure. Within 20 minutes from the start of injection, her blood pressure had returned to normal....from this time on her recovery was uneventful. In this case, urea was definitely life-saving, because prior to its administration, the patient's survival was unlikely. In many similar instances urea was found to be life-saving" (Dr. M. Javid, University of Wisconsin).

Urine: A Billion Dollar Industry

Despite what the public has been led to believe about urine, pharmaceutical companies have grossed billions of dollars from the sale of drugs made from urine constituents. Pergonal, a fertility drug made from human urine, earned a reported $855 million in sales in 1992, and sales ($1400 a month per patient) have increased yearly. Urokinase, a urine ingredient, is used in drug form and sold as a "miracle blood clot dissolver" for unblocking coronary arteries. Urea, medically proven to be one of the best moisturizers in the world has been a boon to cosmetic companies who package it in expensive, glamorized creams and lotions. Ever used Murine ear drops? They're made from carbamide — another name for synthetic urea. When you look at the real facts, the tragedy of the general disinformation campaign on urine is surpassed only by the irony of our unwitting, and often incredibly expensive purchases of what we all mistakenly but firmly believe to be our bodies' "useless" and "offensive" waste-product, urine.

The preceding article was from: **http://all-natural.com/natural-remedies/urine/**

"It's the most astounding proven **natural cure** that medical science has ever discovered-and yet none of the incredible research findings on this incomparable natural medicine have ever been revealed to the public! Now, for the first time ever, learn to use this simple method and read about the startling and amazing medical cures that prestigious researchers and doctors themselves have witnessed in clinical use of this inexpensive, incredibly effective yet virtually unknown natural medicine." This is a summary of the Book: Your Own Perfect Medicine by Martha Christy

My own testimony:

I have used Urine Therapy / Living Water Therapy since June 2013. My entire life has changed as a direct result of consuming my own precious jewels. My skin has a glow and shine that is difficult to explain. People, especially family will tell me over and over again that I look younger and younger each time they see me. This is particularly hard for them to understand because they can clearly see I am without any make-up whatsoever. They are both astonished and amazed.

I did confer with a Naturopathic Doctor before beginning my regimen. The doctor was so excited to share with me that his students are asked to follow the protocol during their studies. Dr. Mark explained of several case studies that had been conducted and how people survived for extended periods of time by existing on nothing more than their own urine. I was fascinated. Mainly because I had never heard of this before now. Knowing there was no harm or danger I never had a repulsive response to the drinking of my own urine. My constitution allows for me to taste and follow protocols that some people claim they cannot. We often accept a pill or other pharmaceutical that is prescribed by a doctor without question. We accept it on blind faith that it will do what the doctor claims. Yet thousands of people are dying each year due to incorrectly prescribed or administered pills. I find that appalling.

I do share but with some reluctance. It has nothing to do with being scared of what these folks will say or how they will respond. I allow my radiant health to be the testimony in and of itself. When asked I proudly explain I consume of my own precious Living Water. I have discussed this topic on my radio show. I drink daily even while away from home on vacation! I never miss a day. Only once did I think it was not a good idea because I was taking some prescription meds. That was only for a brief period of time, maybe a week or so. When I was advised that I could continue without any side effects I immediately resumed my daily dosage. My bare minimum is the first urine of the day. When I feel something going on in my body I increase the intake. At one point I was drinking all that I urinated. I use my living water on my face, in my bath water, on my body and brushing my teeth.

You know what's funny? I receive compliments all the time about my fragrance! People ask me what brand I wear almost daily. I just smile and thank them. So I have allowed experts to summarize and provide information on this vital subject for you. Do as you are directed to do. Follow your spirit and Guidance. However when you are ready just understand that there is absolutely nothing in the whole wide world wrong with YOUR LIVING WATER. It's priceless, valuable, amazing, fortifying and yours free!!

CHAPTER 6

RECIPES

As Nature Intended…

SUPER FOODS

Almonds - Even though almonds are high in fat, they are a way for you to reduce the risk of getting heart disease. They effectively lower your LDL Cholesterol, often referred to as the "bad" cholesterol. Almonds have been credited with helping you feel full when they're added to a meal, helping to gain muscle when combined with weight lifting, and helping to stave off hunger as a snack between meals. Consider using almond butter that contains only almonds if you aren't a fan of chomping up whole nuts.

Apples - Turns out there's a lot of truth in the apple a day adage. Aside from the obvious benefits of containing fiber and helping regular digestive bacteria, apples contain polyphenols that offer an assortment of benefits. The most impressive of which is they're able to help regulate your blood sugar levels, which can be of great use in weight loss, and help you stay focused throughout the day. To get the full benefit, consider spending a bit more for organic rather than conventional. You're leaving out a lot of the toxins and pesticides that get sprayed onto ordinary apples.

Asparagus - The major takeaway on asparagus is that it hits on two levels: it provides antioxidants, and also works as an anti-inflammatory, so you're fighting free radicals and making it easier for your body to maintain its natural state of being.

Avocados - Avocados do contain a decent amount of fat, but it's the good kind of fat, and these can actually help your heart, rather than weigh it down. Guys: these can help with the prevention of prostate cancer. Other top benefits are that it can help prevent other cancers, keep your cholesterol at healthy levels, and help prevent strokes. Useful if you have a family history of stroke.

Bananas - Most of us know that bananas contain a good amount of potassium, but it's also a good source of fiber. When combined, these two features make bananas one of those foods you should try to consume on a daily basis. Why is potassium so important?

It helps to regulate your blood pressure, and this does a great service to your overall heart health, and well-being.

Basil - The flavonoids it contains may help ward off invading cancer cells. There are a lot of recipes that call for basil. With the other ingredients of pesto also being good for you, namely garlic, pine nuts, and extra virgin olive oil, this is a tasty sauce that can break up the marinara routine.

Beans (several kinds) - Beans are getting more and more attention as a good carbohydrate to balance out protein dishes. This is because they don't spike your blood sugar levels like some complex carbs do, and they contain a good amount of fiber. There are plenty of varieties to choose from, such as Kidney beans, Lima beans, Navy beans, Pinto Beans, and the one that's most commonly found: Black beans.

Bell Peppers – Red are best, to get good nutritional value, not just in the form of phytonutrients, but also from Vitamin C, which bell peppers are a surprising source. Green are not ripe. They've also got antioxidants in them that can help you avoid diabetes, and can help you prevent a buildup of cholesterol which can lead to a host of other problems.

Bitter Melon (Ampalaya) – Bitter Melon has strong anti-cancer properties, reverse type-2 diabetes and is a superior holistic care choice. Cooked bitter melon shows significant increase in the free radical scavenging activity versus cold maceration.

Broccoli - Aside from feeling like a giant by eating these tiny trees, broccoli packs a lot into a regular serving. It's got fiber to help with regularity and keeping blood sugar levels optimal, it helps the heart and eyes with lutein, and can help prevent cancer. It's also been shown to help with sun damage, and is good for bones and can help with the nervous system.

Cabbage - Packing more Vitamin C support that the orange, cabbage is a great way to help keep healthy during flu season or anytime of the year. But it doesn't stop there, it also acts to detoxify the body, and can help your brain function at its best. Worried about getting Alzheimer's because it runs in the family? Make sure you get regular cabbage intake.

Carrots - Yes, carrots do actually help with good vision, and they can also help prevent cancer, and they can help slow down the aging process of cells. But that's not all, they've also been shown to help with heart disease, and can have a cleansing effect by providing the liver with Vitamin A so it can do its job better.

Cauliflower - There are plenty of benefits to cauliflower and it makes a great partner to broccoli. They can help prevent cancer, help you digest other foods more easily, and can help with any weight loss efforts. Expecting Moms: This is a good source of folate, so if you've been looking to add more of that to your diet you can count on cauliflower.

Chia Seeds – Chia seeds are a complete protein rich in fiber, potassium, calcium, iron, phosphorus and manganese. Just 1 tablespoon of chia seeds contains 5 grams of fiber.

Coconut – A very healthy saturated fat and perfect for cooking as it is the only oil that stays stable when you heat it. Coconut meat is high in protein and fiber.

Cucumbers - Cucumbers are a good source of water, and while that might sound funny they help to rehydrate the body in a different way than drinking a glass of water does. When preparing them you may be tempted to peel them first since the skin can be hard to chew up, but since it's packed with Vitamin C so you want to leave them on, or at least leave some of it on.

Flax - The fiber in flax is what gets its foot in the superfood door, but it's also packed with omega-3, which you'd usually find in a fish source. Men and women both benefit from its anti-cancer benefits, men with prostate cancer and women with breast cancer. Toss in the evidence showing this can help ward off heart disease, diabetes, and stroke and this is a bona fide winner.

Goji Berries – Gojis are probably one of the most nutritious berry-fruit in the planet. A complete source of protein and amino acids, trace minerals as well as Vitamins B1, B2, B6, E and C. Extremely rich in Anti-oxidants, protects from the aging process and free radicals. They improve vision, boost libido, sexual function and immune system.

Greens - Eat your greens! Many people find them hard to incorporate into a meal, but you can treat them just like spinach in a salad. Collard greens can help detox the body, Mustard greens contain plenty of vitamins and minerals, Turnip greens get you the iron your body needs, Swiss chard can help you with your blood glucose levels, and Kale has carotenoids that make it great for adding to a green smoothie.

Kimchi - This is a staple in Korean cuisine. The most common way it is prepared is with fermented cabbage. It is thought to help aid in digestion the same way that sauerkraut does, by providing digestive enzymes to help us break down the foods we eat more easily.

Kiwi - Whether you go with the standard green variety, or the harder-to-find gold, kiwis are a great source of phytonutrients and fiber, as well as packed with vitamins and minerals. They go great in fruit salads, or they're great by themselves. Eating tip: Cut it in half and spoon it right out of the peel. Fast, easy and yummy!

Lemons and Limes - There are plenty of reasons to start using more lemon and lime in your cooking, or even squeezed into your water. They can help with conditions like indigestion and constipation, and can even be a solution for fevers. Several hair and skin products also contain these natural citrus extracts in them.

Lentils - Lentils often make the list of some of the healthiest foods on the planet. A way to balance out proteins without eating carbs that will make you fat. In addition they've been shown to help with cholesterol levels, heart and digestive health, and giving you a boost of energy.

Mango - If you're already a fan of mango, but find that you don't eat it as often as you'd like to, you might want to find a way to fit it into your cooking repertoire. It can help with things like digestion, the immune system, and even a stagnant libido. If you can't find it fresh when it's not in season, try going the frozen route. Makes a great addition to smoothies.

Miso - Miso is typically presented in soup form, and you may have only experienced it as a side dish to a sushi roll. But it's got you covered as far as amino acids go, and it can even reduce your risk for certain cancers. If you don't like the taste at first, don't give up, as there are several ways to prepare miso soup, and even to use miso paste in other recipes.

Olive Oil - The monounsaturated fatty acids are one good reason to use olive oil if you don't already, because they're heart healthy. The polyphenol content is the next big ace up its sleeve. Use the extra virgin variety for things like salad dressing, and stick to the regular kind if you want to fry foods in it.

Pomegranate - This usually ends up as pomegranate juice, and it makes a great addition to fruit smoothies, or just drinking straight. The top benefits of drinking it are that it can help with breast, prostate, and lung cancer. It's also been shown to help with blood pressure, and can help prevent or even reverse plaque buildup in the arteries.

Mushrooms – **Portobello -** The potassium levels are the first thing that typically gets brought up, but they also contain antioxidants and vegetable based protein for those that don't eat meat. It's often served up as an alternative to a burger, or used in Italian dishes to replace the beef. **Shiitake Mushrooms** - Your immune system can benefit from eating shiitake mushrooms in their whole form. Don't get them confused with the extracts that are used in herbal remedies, as it's not the same. **Reishi Mushroom:** Top cardiovascular healing mushroom. The active ingredient Adenosine removes angina pain, hospitals use it to relive chest pain and normalize irregular heartbeat. Adenosine is a nitrogen rich molecule.

Quinoa - It's got all of the protein you'd want from a super-grain, and it's got plenty of fiber. It also contains plenty of minerals like iron, magnesium, and manganese. Lost on how to prepare it so you can add it to your regular menu? Luckily there are plenty of quinoa recipes to guide the way.

Raisins - As far as antioxidants go, raisins beat out their grape ancestors. They're loaded with tons of other benefits like giving you a burst of energy, and even helping to treat infections. But be careful because there's more sugar in play than with grapes, and it's easier to eat too many raisins and get a sugar rush and subsequent crash.

Sauerkraut - Made from fermented cabbage, sauerkraut adds a lot of flavor to meals but also aids in digestion because of the fermenting process. It acts as a natural probiotic, and it's recommended to eat it before eating the other foods in your meal.

Seeds - Seeds are typically small but can contain a lot of nutrients and healthy benefits depending on what type you eat. **Hemp** seeds can help with different brain functions, eat **Pumpkin** seeds raw for the full sleep-inducing effect, use **Sesame** seeds in dishes like Tahini, **Sunflower** seeds are best when they're eaten raw, and **Chia** seeds have plenty of extra omega-3 in them and can help balance your glucose levels.

Spinach - It might be just as easy to add a spinach salad to your lunch or dinner. The fiber is off the charts, and like many of the other superfoods it helps with blood pressure, immunity, brain function, and has several other benefits.

Sweet Potatoes - They're a good source of iron, as well as magnesium and Vitamin D and C, as well as B6. They're great for reaching weight loss goals and are a good carb.

Tomatoes - There are so many benefits to eating tomatoes that they cover almost every major part of the body including the heart, the skin, and bones. Ward off cancer, fight the harmful effects of smoking, help manage your diabetes, and improve your vision.

Turmeric - Even though it's been around for a long time, turmeric is only recently getting attention as a superfood, or rather super-spice. Add it to the other superfood cauliflower to create a powerful front against prostate cancer. In fact you might want to get into the habit of incorporating this spice into many foods you prepare for its anti-cancer properties.

Walnuts - They say that the brainy look of walnuts is a hint that they're good for the brain, and modern research is backing it up. As long as you follow a healthy diet these can help you keep your mind sharp as you get older. They can also give you a natural energy boost, unlike the energy drinks that get so much attention.

Watermelon - The anti-cancer properties of watermelon are due to the vitamins and antioxidants it contains. It's also a great cooling food for hot summer days, and it's natural sweetness can make this a good food to satisfy your sweet tooth without breaking your diet. Just don't overeat it, as it does contain sugar so keep portion sizes regular.

<u>Interesting nutritional information...</u>

apples	Immune system activator	prevents constipation	Blocks diarrhea	Improves lung capacity	Pectin - Scrubs arteries/ intestines
apricots	Combats cancer	Controls blood pressure	Saves your eyesight	Shields against Alzheimer's	Slows aging process
artichokes	Aids digestion	Lowers cholesterol	Protects your heart	Stabilizes blood sugar	Guards against liver disease
avocados	Liver detox	Lowers cholesterol	Helps stops strokes	Controls blood pressure	Helps with weight loss
bananas	Protects your heart	Quiets a cough	Strengthens bones	Controls blood pressure	Blocks diarrhea
beans	Prevents constipation	Helps hemorrhoids	Lowers cholesterol	Combats cancer	Stabilizes blood sugar
beets	Controls blood pressure	Combats cancer	Strengthens bones	Protects your heart	Aids weight loss
blueberries	Combats cancer	Protects your heart	Stabilizes blood sugar	Boosts memory	Heals eyes and colon
broccoli	Strengthens bones	Saves eyesight	Combats cancer	Promotes liver detox	Controls blood pressure
cabbage	Combats cancer	Prevents constipation	Promotes weight loss	Protects your heart	Repairs stomach and intestinal lining
cantaloupe	Saves eyesight	Controls blood pressure	Lowers cholesterol	Combats cancer	Supports immune system
carrots	Saves eyesight	Protects your heart	Prevents constipation	Combats cancer	Promotes weight loss
cauliflower	Protects against Prostate Cancer	Combats Breast Cancer	Strengthens bones	Banishes bruises	Guards against heart disease
celery	Lowers blood pressure	Raises sex drive	Aides weight loss	Anti-estrogen	High in organic sodium
cherries	Protects your heart	Combats Cancer	Reduces inflammation	Slows aging process	Shields against Alzheimer's
chestnuts	Promotes weight loss	Protects your heart	Lowers cholesterol	Combats Cancer	Controls blood pressure
cilantro	Master of mercury	Autistic help	Helps digestion	Combats Cancer	Heavy metal detox

figs	Promotes weight loss	Helps stops strokes	Lowers cholesterol	Combats Cancer	Controls blood pressure
fish	Protects your heart	Boosts memory	Protects your heart	Combats Cancer	Supports immune system
flax	Aids digestion	Battles diabetes	Protects your heart	Improves mental health	Boosts immune system
garlic	Lowers cholesterol	Controls blood pressure	Combats cancer	Blood thinner	Destroys viruses
grapefruit	Protects against heart attacks	Anti-viral	Helps stops strokes	Cleans arteries, kidneys, liver	Reduces Hepatitis
grapes	saves eyesight	Conquers kidney stones	Combats cancer	Enhances blood flow	Protects your heart
green tea / Organic	Combats cancer	Protects your heart	Helps stops strokes	Promotes Weight loss	Kills bacteria
Honey Manuka	Heals wounds	Aids digestion	Guards against ulcers	Increases energy	Fights allergies
Kale	Optimal Eye, Blood and Bone health	Rebuilds blood	Richest in Chlorophyll, magnesium	Most Vitamin K of any food	Lutein for eye
Kiwi	Reverses Asthma	Lung healing	Vitamin C 2nd highest	Protects from inflammation	Reverses respiratory, allergies and anemic issues
lemons	Combats cancer	Protects your heart	Controls blood pressure	Smooths skin	Stops scurvy
limes	Combats cancer	Protects your heart	Controls blood pressure	Removes uric acid / gout	Inhibits production of HIV
mangoes	Combats cancer	Boosts memory	Regulates thyroid	aids digestion	Shields against Alzheimer's
mushrooms	Controls blood pressure	Lowers cholesterol	Kills bacteria	Combats cancer	Strengthens bones
oats	Lowers cholesterol	Combats cancer	Battles diabetes	prevents constipation	Smooths skin
Okra	Artery scrubber	Colon cleansing	Heart healing	Anti-diabetic	High in soluble fiber
olive oil	Protects your heart	Promotes Weight loss	Combats cancer	Battles diabetes	Smooths skin
onions	Reduce risk of heart attack	Combats cancer	Kills bacteria	Boosts circulation	Prevents blood clots

oranges	Supports immune systems	Combats cancer	Protects your heart	Straightens respiration	Removes uric acid
peaches	prevents constipation	Combats cancer	Helps stops strokes	aids digestion	Helps hemorrhoids
peanuts	Protects against heart disease	Promotes Weight loss	Combats Prostate Cancer	Lowers cholesterol	Aggravates **diverticulitis**
pineapple	Strengthens bones	Anti-cancer	Aids digestion	Pain relief	Better digestion
prunes	Slows aging process	prevents constipation	boosts memory	Lowers cholesterol	Protects against heart disease
quinoa	A complete protein	High fiber	Calcium	Vitamin E	All Essential amino acids
Spinach	Intestinal healing	Chlorophyll and Lutein for eyes	Liver	Constipation remedy	Helps Macular degeneration
strawberries	Anti-cancer protection	Protects your heart	boosts memory	Calms stress	Beauty aide
sweet potatoes	Saves your eyesight	High protein	Combats cancer	Strengthens bones	Low glycemic
tomatoes	Protects prostate	Combats cancer	Lowers cholesterol	Protects your heart	Free radical protection
walnuts	Lowers cholesterol	Combats cancer	Melatonin / Pineal Gland	Maximum brain health	Protects against heart disease
water	Promotes Weight loss	Combats cancer	Conquers kidney stones	Smooths skin	Hydrates body
watermelon	Protects prostate	Promotes Weight loss	Lowers cholesterol	Opens urinary flow	Controls blood pressure

Best Foods for Bone Health

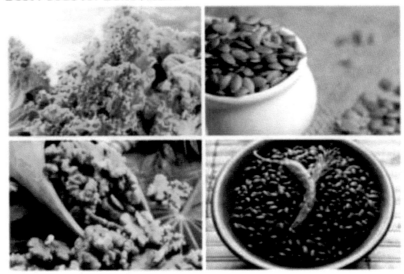

1. Dark Leafy Greens

Dark and leafy, like kale and collard greens pack a one-two-three of calcium, magnesium, and vitamin K. When it comes to strong and healthy bones, these are your #1 for sure. Experiment with other greens like Spinach, Swiss Chard, and Arugula.

2. Seeds

Sprinkle some seeds onto your next salad for some bone-building power. If you want the most bang for your buck, consider mineral-rich pumpkin seeds and sunflower seeds. Soak seeds before using.

3. Nuts

Snack on a handful of nuts to protect your bones. You can add them to soups or salads, use them to top casseroles, or even puree them to make creamy vegan desserts. Want the most bone-protection power?

4. Beans

Beans aren't just a cheap way to round out a meal. They're also packed with nutrients to keep your bones healthy! Black beans in particular are great for building bone health.

Worst Foods for Bone Health

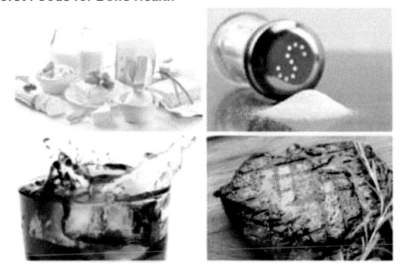

1. Dairy Products

I am as surprised as you are! I knew that dairy wasn't the end all when it comes to bone health, but it turns out that dairy products may leach calcium from bones and increase your risk of fractures over time. What the what?

2. Salt

If you're trying to eat healthily, chances are that you're already cutting out the table salt, and here's one more reason to watch the white stuff: if may increase bone fragility. A Japanese study found that women who ate more salt were four times as likely to fracture a bone.

3. Cola

You may have heard that carbonated beverages or soda pop are bad for your bones, and I found some new research that uncovers what exactly is going on there. Scientists believe that it's actually the phosphoric acid in cola specifically that depletes your bones.

4. Too Much Protein

Healthy eating is all about balance, and of course you need protein to stay healthy, but there's some solid evidence that too much of the stuff can weaken your bones. What's a little bit tricky about this research is that the group who ate less protein also ate a plant-based diet, so it's unclear whether it's the amount of protein or the type of protein that's causing the damage.

"Juicing is the 15 minute nutrient express to health!" - Jason Vale, Hungry For Change

One of the best ways to stay on track with juicing is to learn more about how juicing can benefit your health. Kris Carr, Jason Vale, Mike Adams, Dr. Mercola and Joe Cross in *Hungry For Change* are all passionate advocates of juicing daily and here's their reasons why:

- Juicing allows us to take in a large serving of vegetables and fruits at one time and can be the key to giving you a radiant, energetic life and truly optimal health. Dr. Mercola typically buys up to 20 pounds of raw vegetables per week and juices a few pounds per day. Some people may find eating that many vegetables difficult, but it can be easily accomplished with a quick glass of vegetable juice.

- Juicing is an easy way to absorb all the nutrients from the vegetables. This is important because most of us have impaired digestion as a result of making less-than-optimal food choices over many years. This limits your body's ability to absorb all the nutrients in an optimal way. Juices go straight to your blood stream which in turn carries all the nutrients to where they are needed the most by the body without further delay as in digestion.

- Juicing can help you add a wider variety of vegetables in your diet. Many people eat the same vegetable salads every day. This goes against the principle of regular food rotation and increases your chance of developing an allergy to a certain food. But with juicing, you can juice a wide variety of vegetables that you may not normally enjoy eating whole.

- Juicing is also an incredibly effective way to cleanse the body, especially green juices! Green juices contain high levels of chlorophyll a powerful phytonutrient which attaches to toxins and heavy metals and helps remove them from your body. It also increases your blood's oxygen-carrying capacity by stimulating red blood cell production.

Juicing

Juicing removes the fiber from the vegetables and fruits you are processing. Smoothies, on the other hand includes all the fibers of the fruits and vegetables. You can use the finer from juicing in other recipes as to not lose any nutritional value. With smoothies you retain all the valuable nutrients. I use both methods.

Combinations:

Celery, Lemon and Apple – Alkalizing, better bowel movements and artery scrubber

Celery, Cucumber, Lemon and Apple (Pear) – Lowers BP, Pectin, Strong bones, Skin and cancer protection

Celery, Kale, Lemon, Apple (Pear) – Lutein, Vitamin C, Calcium, Pectin, Chlorophyll, Eye, rebuilds Blood and Bone health

Celery, Lemon, Parsley, Apple (Pear) –Lowers BP, Enhances Sex drive

Celery, Lemon, Fennel, Parsley, Apple – Digestive, Metabolic and Immune System.

These are some easy combinations that you can use. Using these you will find each has the same ingredient of Celery with a few additional items.

Juicing may play an important role in helping you to adjust to a healthier way of eating. Most juicing however removes the pulp from the fruit and vegetable you are juicing. It's relatively easy to enjoy 'freshly prepared juice' store bought juice is often filled with unnecessary sugar, making them high in fructose.

There are multiple recipes and combinations that you can use. Allow your taste to determine the blend that you create. Be careful when it comes to the natural sugars in fruits such as apples, and limit your intake.

SMOOTHIES:

There are so many other health benefits of consuming green smoothie daily. Some of them are:-
• Provides our body with nutrient dense nutrition
• Aids in weight loss
• Boosts energy
• Strengthens the immune system
• Improves overall health and wellness
• Faster healing time
• Lessen cravings for junk type foods.
Many people have cured themselves of all sorts of health problems by incorporating green smoothies into their diet.

Green smoothies are very alkalizing on the body, and an alkaline body is a healthy body. Disease loves an acidic environment, so the more alkalizing food you can eat the better. Smoothies are full of Phytochemicals, vitamins and minerals and good types of carbohydrates. Greens are full of chlorophyll straight from the sun boosting your nutrition for optimum health and wellbeing.

This is up to you really. You might want to start off with around 25% greens until you get used to it and then slowly build that up to as much as you like. Ideally if you are doing a 1 liter smoothie you should be looking at about the equivalent of 1 head of lettuce or more. The amount of water is also up to you. Some people like a thick soupy smoothie that you might even choose to eat like a pudding while other people like it thin and watery. Keep in mind though if you are going to make it a thin consistency you will probably want to make more overall so you can still get a good amount of fruits and greens in.

A glass or two a day is perfect for adding important nutrients to your daily diet. You can either drink the whole thing as an entire meal or split it into a couple of smaller smoothies to drink during the day. Like everything moderation is the key. A green smoothie is a meal replacement or added extra to your daily diet. You still need to eat other 'real' foods as well.

Watch the fruit intake Just make sure not to overdo it on the fruit as it is now recommended for health that it is wise to limit fruit fructose to 25 grams or less per day.

However for someone that is overweight or has health issues it would actually be wise to limit your fruit fructose to 15 grams or less. This is not much – it represents two bananas, one third cup raisins or just two Medjool dates. You will get more as it virtually guaranteed you will consume 'hidden' sources of fructose from most beverages or just about any processed food.

SMOOTHIES

Allow your imagination to assist you in the making of your morning drink. Here are recommended proportions, Build to suit your taste and preference.

Water	Ionized Alkaline or distilled	2 cups
Greens	Chard, Arugula, Spinach, Kale, Spring Mix, Romaine	1 ½ cups
Avocado		½
Apple	Organic	½
Sprouts	Sunflower, Lentil, Mung, Buckwheat, (can use more than 1)	¼ cup
Goji Berries		1 Tablespoon
Chia, Sesame, Flax		1 Tablespoon
Himalayan Sea Salt		1 Teaspoon
Dulce		2 teaspoons

May add:
Banana
Strawberry
Blue Berries
Blackberries
Pineapple
Mango
Pear

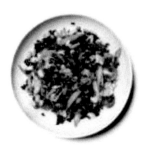

Black Rice Salad with Lemon Vinaigrette

The pleasantly earthy flavor of black rice pairs well with the bright acidity of this vinaigrette. If you can't find it, use wild rice instead. 6 servings

Active: 15 minutes Total: 1 hour 20 minutes

Recipe by Lake Austin Spa Resort in Austin, TX

Ingredients

- 1 cup black rice (preferably Lotus Foods Forbidden Rice)
- Kosher salt
- 1/2 cup walnuts
- 1/4 cup Meyer lemon juice or 3 tablespoons regular lemon juice
- 2 tablespoons white wine vinegar
- 1 tablespoon agave syrup (nectar) or honey
- 1/4 cup extra-virgin olive oil
- 4 scallions, thinly sliced
- 1 cup frozen shelled edamame, thawed
- 1 cup grape tomatoes, halved
- 4 ounces green beans, thinly sliced (about 1 cup)
- Freshly ground black pepper

Preparation

- Preheat oven to 350°. Cook rice in a medium saucepan of boiling salted water until tender, 35-40 minutes. Drain well, spread out on a plate or a rimmed baking sheet, and let cool.
- Meanwhile, spread out walnuts on another rimmed baking sheet. Toast in oven, tossing once, until fragrant, 8-10 minutes. Let cool; chop.
- Whisk lemon juice, vinegar, and agave in a small bowl. Whisking constantly, gradually drizzle in oil. Season vinaigrette with salt.
- Toss rice, walnuts, scallions, edamame, tomatoes, green beans, and vinaigrette in a large bowl. Season with salt and pepper.

- **Nutritional Information:** 6 servings, 1 serving contains: Calories (kcal) 310 , Fat (g) 18, Saturated Fat (g) 2, Cholesterol (mg) 0, Carbohydrates (g) 35, Dietary Fiber (g) 4,
  Total Sugars (g) 5, Protein (g) 8, Sodium (mg) 110

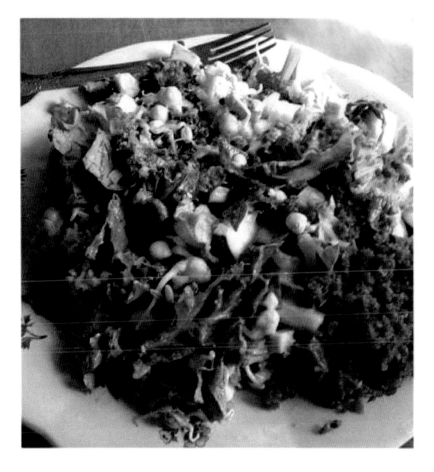

Sandy Salad – an everyday staple

Fresh greens – Romaine, Chard, Collard, Kale, Arugula, Mixed or Spring mix
Fresh sprouts – Garbanzos, sunflower, lentil, mong
Organic cucumber
Organic Avocado
Carrots or celery or zucchini or broccoli
Seasoned with Himalayan sea salt, cayenne pepper and Dulse (sea vegetable)
Dressing – lemon juice or organic virgin olive oil mixed with Apple Cider Vinegar
Add a side of Veggie Kraut

- **Kale and Quinoa Salad 3 Ways**
- Yield: 2 servings
-
- 1/2 bunch curly or purple kale (about 6 leaves), thick stems removed, cut into thin strips (1 cup)
- 2 teaspoons fresh lemon juice
- 1 teaspoon extra-virgin olive oil
- pinch salt
- 1/4 cup cashews, soaked and chopped
- 1/4 cup raisins
- 1 1/2 cups cooked quinoa (see recipe below)
- fresh ground black pepper (optional)
-
- Put the kale, lemon juice, oil, and salt in a medium bowl. Toss well with your hands, working the dressing into the greens. Add the cashews, raisins, and quinoa and toss to combine. Season with fresh ground pepper if desired. Stored in a sealed container in the refrigerator, Kale and Quinoa Salad will keep for 3 days.
-
- **Variations:**
- 1. For Kale Salad with Olives and Bell Peppers: Omit the raisins. Add 1/2 diced red bell pepper and 2 tablespoons sliced black olives along with the cashews and quinoa.
- 2. For Kale Salad with Avocados and Tomatoes: Omit the olive oil, and massage the greens with just the lemon juice and salt. Then add 1/2 diced avocado and massage gently, working the avocado into the greens. Replace the cashews and raisins with 1 diced tomato or 8 quartered cherry tomatoes. This variation should be served within 12 hours.
- **Basic Quinoa**
- Yield: 3 cups, 4 servings
-
- 1 cup quinoa
- 1 3/4 cups water
- Pinch salt
-
- Put the quinoa, water, and salt in a medium saucepan, cover, and bring to a boil. Turn down the heat to low, and cook until all the water is absorbed, about 15 minutes. Turn off the heat and let sit for 5 minutes before serving.
-
- Alternatively, put the quinoa, water, and salt in a rice cooker and turn on. It will take approximately 20 minutes to cook.
-
- Stored in a sealed container in the refrigerator, cooked quinoa will keep for 5 days. It will keep in the freezer for one month.
- --
-
- Now here's something to think about as you're enjoying your salad: kale is full of vitamins, micronutrients, and it also provides calcium, protein, and omega-3 fatty acids.

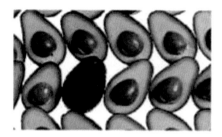

I simply LOVE avocados. I eat at least 1 every day. As a young person I did not know the health benefit and refused to taste them. NOW I cannot go a day without one!!! They are very healthy.

Avocados are one of our most versatile foods.

They can be a great weight loss tool but you want to enjoy them in moderation. The fat in avocados are the "good kind."

They are high in omega 3 fatty acids, which reduce cholesterol and cut the risk of heart disease. Each cup of avocado contains about 3 grams of protein and very little sugar. It also is high in vitamins K, vitamin B5, magnesium, phosphorus, and iron.

FACT: Avocados contain more potassium per gram than bananas.

Besides being good for your heart, avocados are healthy in many other ways.

- They reduce inflammation and regulate blood sugar.

- They control blood pressure, improve vision and strengthen the immune system.

- Their high fiber keeps your digestive system on track and keep you feeling full longer.

- Plus, the high levels of vitamin C and vitamin E that they contain are excellent for your skin.

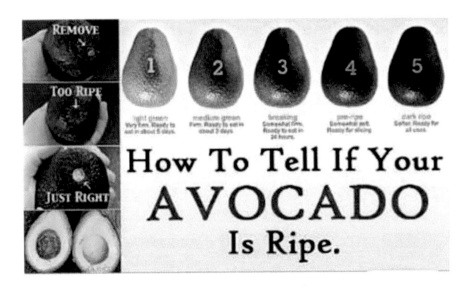

How To Tell If Your AVOCADO Is Ripe.

Four A's Salad (Avocado, Apple, Arugula, Asparagus)

INGREDIENTS

1 avocado

1 apple

1 bunch asparagus

4 cups arugula

3 T extra virgin olive oil

3 T fresh squeezed orange juice

1 tsp honey

DIRECTIONS

Toss asparagus in 1 T. olive oil and roast in 450 degree oven 'til browned.
Remove from oven and allow to cool, then chop into two inch pieces.
Whisk together remaining olive oil, orange juice and honey or agave and set aside.
Chop apple into 1/2-inch pieces, peel and dice avocado into ½-inch cubes.
Put arugula in large bowl and add apple, avocado and asparagus pieces, then mix in salad dressing.

Vitamin Water

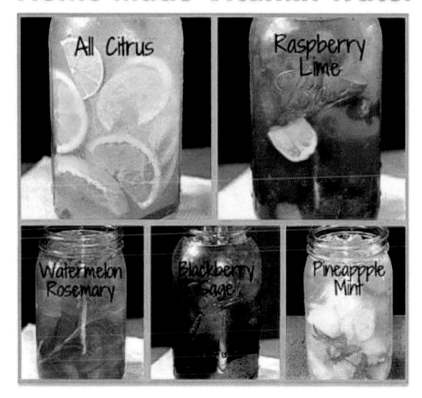

Make your own vitamin water. Add fruits instead of sugar for a natural sweetener for your H20. Cut the fruit into paper-thin slices or small chunks. Combine ingredients with water. Refrigerate 4-6 hours and serve over ice. So delicious and very refreshing!

Black Bean Mango Salsa

1 Cup Black Beans – Freshly prepared

1 large Mango – peeled and chopped, about 2 cups

½ Lime – juiced

½ Medium Red Pepper – chopped

1 Jalapeno Pepper – Chopped, optional, use a dash of hot sauce

1 Medium Scallion or 3 Tablespoons chopped onions

1 Tablespoon Olive Oil

1 ½ teaspoon Rice Wine or Balsamic Vinegar

1 ½ Tablespoon Fresh Ginger – grated

1 Pinch of Cayenne Pepper

1 Tablespoon Fresh Cilantro, chopped

½ teaspoon Himalayan Sea Salt

Mix and refrigerate – serve with organic chips or vegetables

KALE SALAD

Kale	1 bunch Organic, cut into ½" strips
Lemon	½ lemon juiced
Cilantro	1 cup, chopped fine
Avocado	2 medium, chunked
Onion	½ cup chopped
Garlic	5-6 cloves minced
Tomato	2 Roma chopped
Olive oil	2 Tablespoons
Seasonings:	
Cayenne Pepper	1 Tablespoon (to your taste)
Himalayan Sea Salt	1 teaspoon

Rub the olive oil into the Kale to soften. Work the lemon juice into the Kale and let stand for several hours.

Mix all the ingredients together. Refrigerate for 2 hours and serve.

Sautéed Kale

Organic Kale	1 bunch
Garlic	6-8 cloves
Red Onion	1 Medium
Sun-dried Tomatoes	8-10 Pieces
Red Bell pepper	1 Medium – Organic
Cayenne Pepper	1 teaspoon + to suit your taste
Himalayan Sea Salt	1 teaspoon
Coconut Oil	2 Tablespoons

Serve over Quinoa

Directions:
Soak tomatoes 4-6 hours and chop into small pieces
Rinse Kale in vinegar/acid water wash
Cut Kale into 1" strips
Chop garlic, onions, and bell peppers
In a large pot, sauté in Organic Coconut oil the onions, garlic and bell peppers for 3-4 minutes on medium high temp, lower to medium
Add Kale and let simmer 3 additional minutes, as it cooks down add another handful of Kale
Stir to mix from the bottom
Season to taste

Kale will be soften in about 5 minutes
Remove from heat
And In-joy served over Quinoa

Spicy Kale

Kale	1 bunch green or red, cut in ½" pieces
Onion	1 cup red or green, chopped
Garlic	6-8 cloves, minced
Peppers	6-8 peppers chopped
Sun-dried Tomatoes	8-10 pieces, soaked 4-6 hours
Nutritional Yeast	1 Tablespoon
Avocado	2 medium, diced or cubed
Cayenne Pepper	1 Tablespoon
Himalayan Sea Salt	1 teaspoon
Olive Oil	2 Tablespoons

Directions:

Mix Kale with olive oil and let stand for 1 hour.

Drain water from tomatoes.

Chop all ingredients and mix together.

Season to taste and serve in a lettuce or collard green leaf or spinach tortilla.

QUINOA SALAD

Quinoa	2 cups (uncooked)
Red Onion	1 cup
Lime juice	6 Tablespoons
Black Beans	3 cups cooked
Corn	2 cups (fresh or frozen)
Tomatoes	6 Roma
Jalapeno Pepper	3
Cilantro	1 cup
Olive Oil	9 Tablespoons
Goat Cheese	15 oz.

Seasonings:
Cayenne
Himalayan Sea Salt

Directions:

Cook black beans and set aside to cool.

Prepare Quinoa and let cool.

Chop all of the ingredients – onion, tomatoes, jalapeno peppers, cilantro and mix together.

In a large bowl, combine quinoa, black beans and corn mix together.

Add the chopped ingredients, mix in the lime juice, olive oil and goat cheese.

Season to taste and serve.

GOJI BERRY NUTELLA CHIA PUDDING

Coconut milk	1 cup
Honey or Grade B maple syrup	2 teaspoons
Cacao Powder	1 Tablespoon
Pure Vanilla extract	½ teaspoon
Himalayan Sea Salt	pinch
Chia Seeds	5 Tablespoons
Goji Berries	4 Tablespoons
Nuts (Hazel, almonds, pistachio)	4 Tablespoons chopped

Directions:

Mix milk, honey, cacao, vanilla and salt together in a blender until smooth. Remove and place in a bowl.

Stir in the chia seeds, goji berries, and nuts.

Pour into smaller serving size dishes.

Refrigerate at least 20 minutes before serving.

Great for a breakfast replacement.

Very fulfilling and nutritious.

FROZEN DESSERT
(NO DIARY)

Bananas	4 Large, frozen
Frangelico Liqueur	½ cup
Almond Butter	½ cup

Blend all ingredients together in a blender until thoroughly mixed and smooth.

Optional: Serve sliced almonds on top.

RED CABBAGE AND MANGO SLAW

Recipes: http://nutritionstudies.org/recipes/salad/

INGREDIENTS:

Red Cabbage	2 cups shredded
Carrots	2 cups, peeled and chopped or shredded
Mango	1 diced
Cilantro	½ cup chopped (or to taste)
Lime	1 medium juiced, freshly squeezed
Vinegar	Balsamic, to taste
Himalayan Sea Salt	Sprinkle (optional)

PREPARATION:

1. In a large bowl, mix together cabbage, carrots, mango and cilantro. Add lime juice, balsamic vinegar and salt (if using) and toss completely. Taste for seasonings and adjust if needed.
2. Allow slaw to chill completely and mix again very well just before serving.

BAKED SWEET POTATO STICKS

INGREDIENTS:

Sweet Potatoes   1 lb. cleaned and sliced

Olive Oil   2 Tablespoons

Himalayan Sea Salt   pinch, to your taste

DIRECTIONS:

1. Preheat oven to 400 degrees F.
2. Cut the potatoes into sticks lengthwise. Place potato sticks in a bowl with the olive oil and salt. Toss to coat the potatoes.
3. Place potato sticks on a baking sheet and bake for 20-25 minutes or until the fries are crisp and golden on the outside and tender on the inside. Enjoy!!

- Perfect as a replacement for French fries
- Get all the power-food benefits
- Great of gatherings, excellent crowd pleaser

Salads, Meals, Suggestions

Salads

Greens	- Romaine, Mixed Greens, Spinach, Chard, Arugula, or Kale	
Red Bell Pepper		
Avocado		
Sprouts	Mung, Sunflower, Lentil,	
Veggie Kraut	Optional (Probiotics,	
Salad Dressing	Olive oil and Apple Cider Vinegar	
Seasoning	Cayenne pepper, Himalayan sea salt	

Meals: never be afraid to experiment with different ideas. Here are some I have created.

1. Quinoa – mixed with Okra, Red Bell pepper, Sweet potato, Onion, Basil and Garlic. Cook Quinoa according to directions. Chop all veggies. Combine all ingredients together. Season to taste.
2. Zucchini, garlic, carrots, celery and soaked Chickpeas.
3. Mix your favorite veggies together. Season to taste. ENJOY!!

SHOPPING LIST

DIRTY DOZEN – BUY ORGANIC ONLY	CLEAN 15
Apples	Onions
Celery	Avocado
Tomatoes	Sweet Corn
Cucumbers	Pineapple
Grapes	Mango
Nectarines	Sweet Peas
Peaches	Eggplant
Potatoes	Cauliflower
Spinach	Asparagus
Strawberries	Kiwi
Blueberries	Cabbage
Sweet Bell Peppers	Watermelon * seeded
Green Beans	Grapefruit
Kale	Sweet Potatoes
Snap Peas	Honeydew Melon
Hot Peppers	

Definition:

Dirty Dozen – only purchase organic items. These foods can absorb the toxins easily into the meat of the vegetable/fruit.

Clean 15 – It is not necessary to limit these to organic only.

Recommendation – Purchase organic as often as possible.

CHAPTER 7

RESOURCES

WHERE TO GO

We live in an abundant Universe where help and resources are readily available to us to assist with any help or information we may require. We give Thanks to live in such a World that feeds us with what we desire.

DVD's

Here is a <u>partial listing</u> of valuable DVD's that you may want to add to your library.

- ♥ **Doctored**
- ♥ **Fed Up**
- ♥ **Eating – 3rd Edition**
- ♥ **Hungry for Change**
- ♥ **Food Matters**
- ♥ **Greens Can Save Your Life – 1 and 2 by Victoria Boutenko**
- ♥ **Open Sesame**
- ♥ **Dead Wrong – The Film**
- ♥ **Fat, Sick and Nearly Dead**
- ♥ **Fresh – The Movie**
- ♥ **May I Be Frank?**
- ♥ **Genetic Roulette**
- ♥ **The Beautiful Truth**
- ♥ **Fresh**
- ♥ **The Marketing of Madness**
- ♥ **The Tapping Solution**
- ♥ **Doctor Yourself**
- ♥ **Bought**
- ♥ **The Truth About Cancer**
- ♥ **Healing Cancer from the Inside Out**
- ♥ **Eating**

Some excerpts from Food Matters DVD

"You cannot 'heal' one thing and not 'heal' the whole body" Charlotte Gerson. "You cannot 'heal' selectivity, if you truly heal everything heals!" (My emphasis with the exclamation mark)

Journal of American Medical Association –
106 Thousand Americans die from deaths directly associated with their prescribed pharmaceuticals each year.
Adverse drug reaction kills 10 thousand;
Auto accidents kill 3.5 thousand and
Prostate Cancer kills 9 thousand!!
These numbers are staggering when you look at how many are dying from prescribed drugs!!

Drug companies are <u>NOT</u> required to publish their failed trials.

Cancer Research -
President Nixon initiated the 'war on cancer' by allocating $300 million yearly, total funded $39 billion dollars for research. Twenty five years later 569,000 people have died, doubled that from original onset.

Conclusion = Best Doctor, Best Nutritionist = **YOU!!!**

Some excerpts from BOUGHT DVD

Environmental triggers causes genetic mutation/Autism.

The three big or BIG 3 Corporations in America = Drug, Vaccine, Food, total $30 billion yearly revenue.

In 1996 GMO/GEO were introduced, all dis-eases have increased since 1996!!!

Vaccines – HPV and flu vaccines no research done on either!!
HPV no clinical trials performed and it contains huge amounts of aluminum!
Flu – no research and no more effective than anything else which has been proven. Pregnant women suffer fetal deaths after getting the vaccine.

FOOD = MEDICINE
Paleo Diet – A SCIENTIFIC PERSPECTIVE by Brenda Davis

These are my notes from the lecture by Brenda Davis. I am listing the most significant facts that she presented in my view.

Red meat and Mortality
Consumption of red meat had these health consequences on humans
- ⇒ Increased 25%+ of death (3oz.)
- ⇒ Increased risk of diabetes 50% (3oz.)
- ⇒ All cancers – 10-25% increased, processed meat = 20-30%
- ⇒ WHO – World Health Organization has listed processed and red meat as a carcinogenic

Chicken – lead contaminants in broth
Bone broth – no research on benefits to human health

I cite these as examples that we must be vigilant and educate ourselves on the contents of the things we ingest believing that it is a natural product. So much has changed, so many have and are manipulating organisms in the laboratory and marketing the items as food! So much of what we have in our markets and grocery stores is **NOT** food.

These manufacturers that I am writing about now have caused a disruption in the eco-system of our planet. AND the cross-breeding of unnatural species is having a direct effect on our overall health and the quality of our lifestyles.

Our children suffer the most. For many of them have never eaten real, whole foods. The school system is a part of the whole process of feeding our babies things that do more harm than good to their bodies.

The Diary Industry in particular reasonable for marketing their products as if we cannot survive without them. All the while knowing from research that cow's milk causes a multitude of health concerns especially for the children and girls! With a clear conscious and pure intent how can they promote a product that is not intended for human consumption? Cow's milk is for baby cows or calves. The nutrients in the milk is to afford tremendous growth for the calf. A calf grows from 60 pounds to 600 pounds and the mother's milk is created to provide for that growth. So is it any wonder why our girls especially are forming and maturing their little bodies so early in life. It could be in the milk!!

I am just saying, there has to be a time when we no longer blindly follow the suggestions of an apparently biased system of greed and corruption. Is it really for our benefit? And if so, where is the profit margin for the corporations? Simply asking you to think.

OTHER RESOURCES:

Dr. Mark Armstrong	www.ahimki.net
Ty Bollinger	www.thetruthaboutcancer.com
Dr. T. Colin Campbell	www.nutritionstudies.org
Jeffrey Smith	www.responsibletechnology.org
(IRT - INSTITUTE for RESPONSIBLE TECHNOLOGY)	
Dr. Joseph Mercola	www.Mercola.com
Jeff Primack	www.qirevolution.com
Carla DeRosa	www.rawxit.com
Care2 Healthy Living	www.care2.com
Organics Consumers Associations	www.organicconsumers.org
Food Matters	www.foodmatters.tv
Reboot with Joe Blog	www.rebootwithjoe.com
Consumers for Dental Choice	www.toxicteeth.org
Mercury Free Dentists	www.mercuryfreedentists.com

Jeff Hayes – Bought	www.jeffhaysfilms.com
Sacred Science (For elders)	www.thesacredscience.com
Dr. Cayce	www.cayce.com
Pedram Shojai, Well.org	www.well.org
Jordan Reasoner (Gluten)	www.scdlifestyle.com
Ocean Robbins	www.foodrevolution.org
Dr. Tom O'Bryan (Gluten)	www.thedr.com
Urine Therapy	http://www.urinetherapy.in/CaseHistory.aspx
	http://all-natural.com/natural-remedies/urine/
Dr. Garry Gordon	www.gordonresearch.com
Brenda Cobb	http://www.livingfoodsinstitute.com
Living Foods Institute	www.livingfoodsinstitute.com
Ann Wigmore's Story –	www.http://hippocratesinst.org
GA. Farmers Market Association	www.mygeorgiamarket.org
Wholesome Wave	www.WholesomeWave.Org
Dr. John McDougall	www.drmcdugall.com
Dr. Christiane Northrup	www.drnorthrup.com
Dr. William Richardson	www.acpm.net

Atlanta Eateries:

Tassili's Raw Reality   **1059 Ralph D. Abernathy Blvd, SW Atlanta 30310 / 404-343-6126**
www.tassilisraw.com

Lov'N It Live   **2796 East Point St, East Point GA 404-765-9220**
www.lovingitlive.com

R. Thomas   **1812 Peachtree Street, Atlanta GA 30309 404-881-0246**
www.rthomasdeluxegrill.net

Café Sunflower   **2140 Peachtree St NW, Atlanta, GA 30309 / 404-352-8859**
www.cafesunflower.com

Wet My Whistle   **1750 Powder Springs Road, Suite 290 Marietta GA 30064 / 770-821-8314**
WWW.wet-my-whistle.com

NATURAL WONDERS

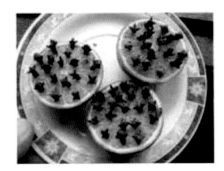

Have a mosquito problem??? At your next outdoor gathering try this SAFE and EFFECTIVE method of keeping mosquitoes at bay! Simply slice a lime in half and press in a good amount of cloves for an ALL NATURAL mosquito repellent... Make sure to SHARE THIS with your friends!

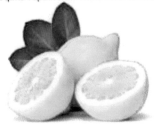

* Keep Out Kitty. What smells great to humans is repulsive to cats. Adding some lemon juice to a spray bottle, and misting an off-limits area — like the kitchen countertops, for instance, or the Christmas tree — will help keep feisty felines away.

* Breathe New Life Into a Humidifier. If your humidifier is starting to smell a little strange, just add a few teaspoons (3-4) to the water.

* Kill Weeds Naturally. Lemon juice is an ultra-effective weed killer. Soak the unwanted plants with the stuff to kill them without all of the harsh chemicals.

* Revive Hardened Paintbrushes. Give a new life to those hardened bristles. Bring lemon juice to a boil on the stove, drop in the brushes, and let it sit for about 15 minutes. Wash and rinse in soap water and let dry.

* Repel Ants and Other Pests. Ants, roaches, and moths hate the smell of citrus. Place lemon juice in a spray bottle, and regularly mist door thresholds, window sills, and anywhere else bugs might creep in.

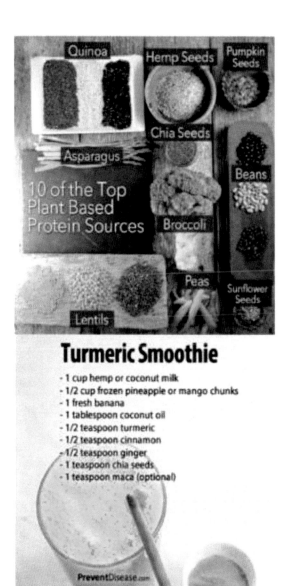

Turmeric Smoothie

- 1 cup hemp or coconut milk
- 1/2 cup frozen pineapple or mango chunks
- 1 fresh banana
- 1 tablespoon coconut oil
- 1/2 teaspoon turmeric
- 1/2 teaspoon cinnamon
- 1/2 teaspoon ginger
- 1 teaspoon chia seeds
- 1 teaspoon maca (optional)

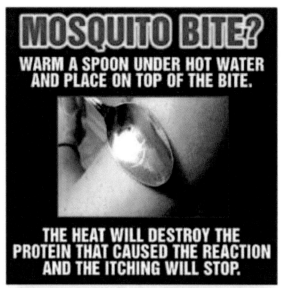

MOSQUITO BITE?

WARM A SPOON UNDER HOT WATER AND PLACE ON TOP OF THE BITE.

THE HEAT WILL DESTROY THE PROTEIN THAT CAUSED THE REACTION AND THE ITCHING WILL STOP.

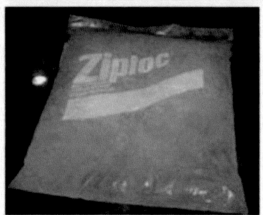

I tell all my patients this at physical therapy! Homemade Ice packs: 1 part rubbing alcohol to 3 parts water, gets really cold, but never hardens so you can manipulate it. every athlete (or mom) should pin this!

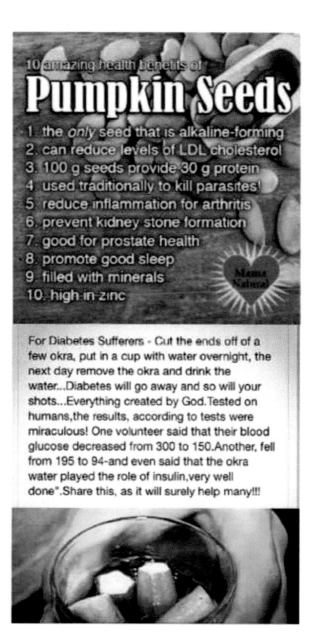

10 amazing health benefits of

Pumpkin Seeds

1. the *only* seed that is alkaline-forming
2. can reduce levels of LDL cholesterol
3. 100 g seeds provide 30 g protein
4. used traditionally to kill parasites!
5. reduce inflammation for arthritis
6. prevent kidney stone formation
7. good for prostate health
8. promote good sleep
9. filled with minerals
10. high in zinc

Mama Natural

For Diabetes Sufferers - Cut the ends off of a few okra, put in a cup with water overnight, the next day remove the okra and drink the water...Diabetes will go away and so will your shots...Everything created by God. Tested on humans, the results, according to tests were miraculous! One volunteer said that their blood glucose decreased from 300 to 150. Another, fell from 195 to 94-and even said that the okra water played the role of insulin, very well done". Share this, as it will surely help many!!!

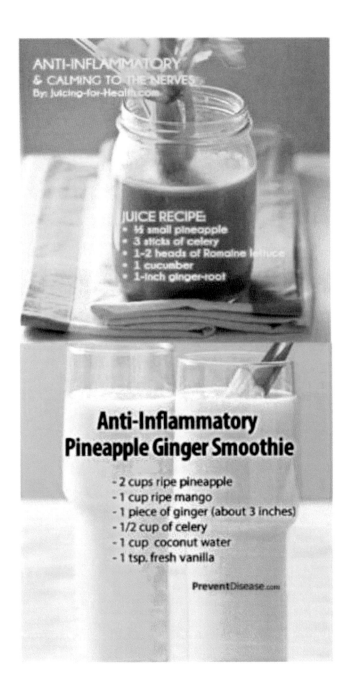

ANTI-INFLAMMATORY
& CALMING TO THE NERVES
By: Juicing-for-Health.com

JUICE RECIPE:
- ½ small pineapple
- 3 sticks of celery
- 1-2 heads of Romaine lettuce
- 1 cucumber
- 1-inch ginger-root

Anti-Inflammatory Pineapple Ginger Smoothie

- 2 cups ripe pineapple
- 1 cup ripe mango
- 1 piece of ginger (about 3 inches)
- 1/2 cup of celery
- 1 cup coconut water
- 1 tsp. fresh vanilla

PreventDisease.com

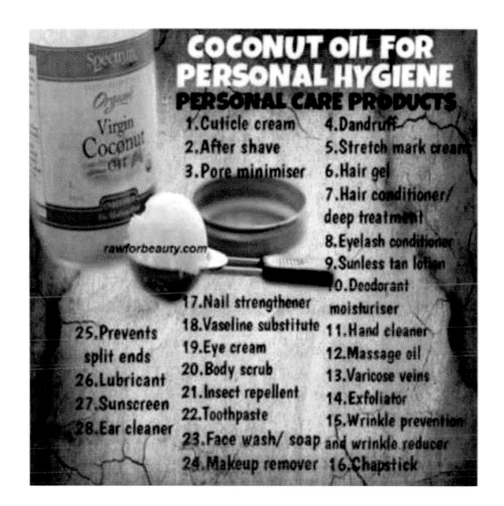

COCONUT OIL FOR PERSONAL HYGIENE
PERSONAL CARE PRODUCTS

1. Cuticle cream
2. After shave
3. Pore minimiser
4. Dandruff
5. Stretch mark cream
6. Hair gel
7. Hair conditioner/ deep treatment
8. Eyelash conditioner
9. Sunless tan lotion
10. Deodorant moisturiser
11. Hand cleaner
12. Massage oil
13. Varicose veins
14. Exfoliator
15. Wrinkle prevention and wrinkle reducer
16. Chapstick
17. Nail strengthener
18. Vaseline substitute
19. Eye cream
20. Body scrub
21. Insect repellent
22. Toothpaste
23. Face wash/ soap
24. Makeup remover
25. Prevents split ends
26. Lubricant
27. Sunscreen
28. Ear cleaner

rawforbeauty.com

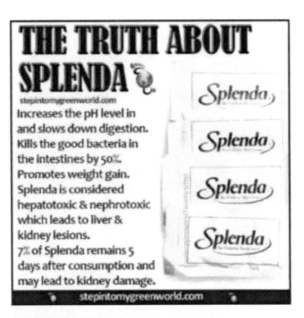

THE TRUTH ABOUT SPLENDA

stepintomygreenworld.com

Increases the pH level in and slows down digestion. Kills the good bacteria in the intestines by 50%. Promotes weight gain. Splenda is considered hepatotoxic & nephrotoxic which leads to liver & kidney lesions. 7% of Splenda remains 5 days after consumption and may lead to kidney damage.

stepintomygreenworld.com

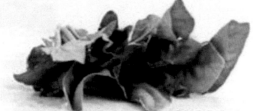

Chlorophyll is plant blood · Almost identical to our own red blood cells · Cleanses the blood · Binds with heavy metals and helps remove them from the body · Cleanses the bowel Increases red blood cell count · Oxygenates the blood Alkalises the blood · Helps fight disease · Strengthens immunity Anti-inflammatory · Antioxidant · Cancer protective

CHLOROPHYLL

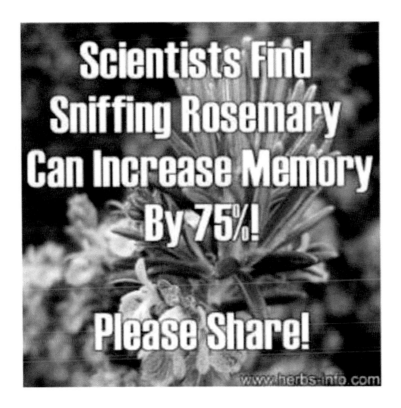

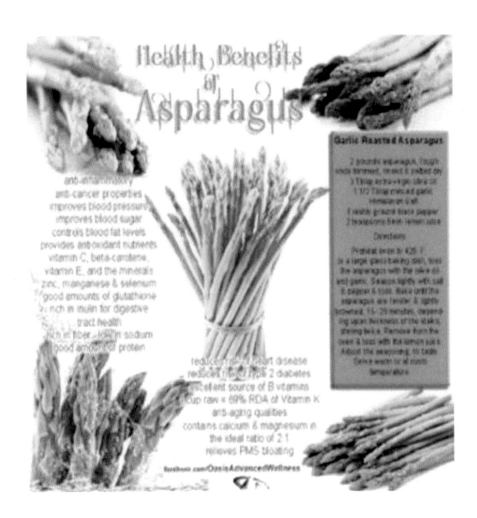

AS NATURE INTENDED

GOD DESIGNED LIFE TO BE SIMPLE...Rev. Sandy Rodgers

GOD's GROCERIES
Facebook: God's Groceries...as Nature Intended
Blogs: revsandy.wordpress.com

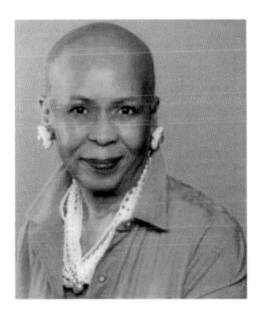

SANDY RODGERS MINISTRIES INC

Stay connected: SRM@SandyRodgersMinistries.org
www.SandyRodgersMinistries.org
P.O. Box 67, Austell GA 30168
404-307-2983

LIFE LOVE WELLNESS
THE SANDY RODGERS SHOW
Every Tuesday 9pm EST / 6pm PST
Accessible wherever you are....
Online: www.blogtalkradio.com/SandyRodgers
or call in 516-531-9819

SANDY RODGERS AUTHENTIC ASCENSION
sandy@SRAuthenticAscension.com
www.SRAuthenticAscension.com

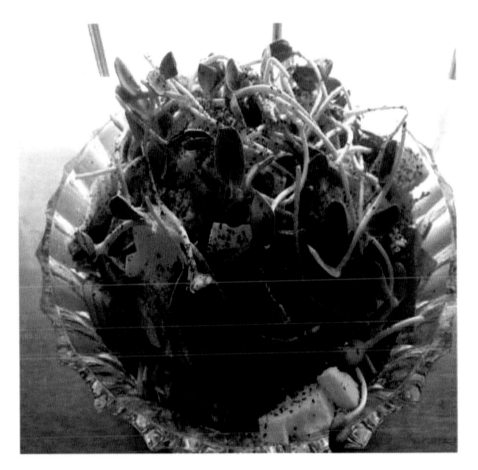

TO YOUR HEALTH!!!
EAT CLEAN

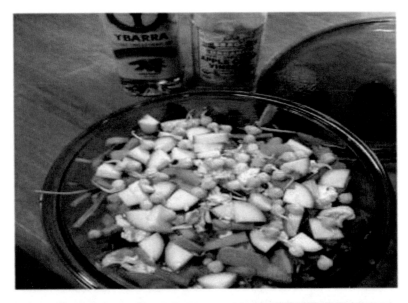

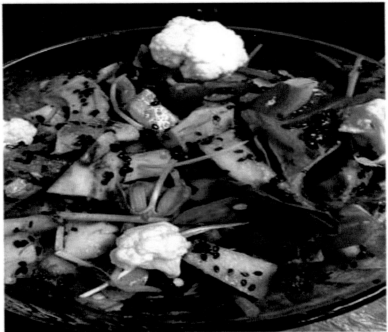

EAT THE RAINBOW – DELICIOUSNESS